S0-EAS-691

Teen Health Series

Complementary And Alternative Medicine Information For Teens, Third Edition

Teen Health Series

Complementary And Alternative Medicine Information For Teens, Third Edition

Health Tips About Diverse Medical And Wellness Systems

Including Information About Chiropractic Medicine And Other Manipulative Practices, Movement And Massage Therapies, Yoga And Other Mind-Body Therapies, Acupuncture And Other Forms Of Energy Medicine, Creative Arts Therapies, And More

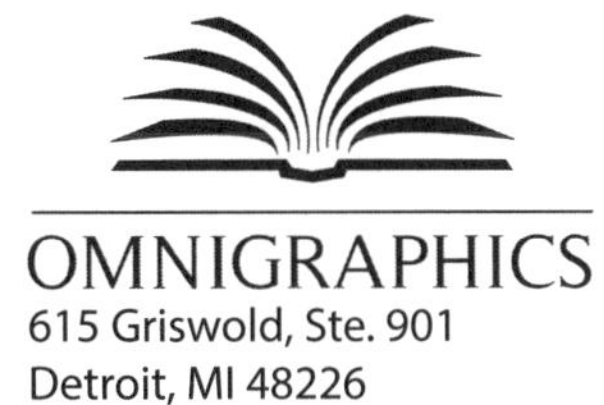

OMNIGRAPHICS
615 Griswold, Ste. 901
Detroit, MI 48226

Bibliographic Note

Because this page cannot legibly accommodate all the copyright notices, the Bibliographic Note portion of the Preface constitutes an extension of the copyright notice.

* * *

OMNIGRAPHICS
John Tilly, *Managing Editor*

* * *

ISBN 978-0-7808-1617-6
E-ISBN 978-0-7808-1618-3

Library of Congress Cataloging-in-Publication Data

Names: Omnigraphics, Inc., issuing body.

Title: Complementary and alternative medicine information for teens: health tips about diverse medical and wellness systems including information about chiropractic medicine and other manipulative practices, movement and massage therapies, yoga and other mind-body therapies, acupuncture and other forms of energy medicine, creative arts therapies, and more.

Description: Third edition. | Detroit, MI: Omnigraphics, Inc., [2018] | Series: Teen health series | Audience: Grade 9 to 12. | Includes bibliographical references and index.

Identifiers: LCCN 2017057394 (print) | LCCN 2017059397 (ebook) | ISBN 9780780816183 (eBook) | ISBN 9780780816176 (hardcover: alk. paper)

Subjects: LCSH: Alternative medicine--Popular works. | Teenagers--Health and hygiene--Popular works.

Classification: LCC R733 (ebook) | LCC R733.C6556 2018 (print) | DDC 610.835--dc23

LC record available at https://lccn.loc.gov/2017057394

This book is printed on acid-free paper meeting the ANSI Z39.48 Standard. The infinity symbol that appears above indicates that the paper in this book meets that standard.

Printed in the United States

Table Of Contents

Part Four: Mind-Body Medicine

Part Five: Biologically Based Practices

Part Six: Energy Medicine

Part Seven: Creative Arts Therapies

Part Eight: CAM Treatments For Cancer And Other Diseases And Conditions

Part Nine: If You Need More Information

Preface

About This Book

The National Center for Complementary and Integrative Health (NCCIH) defines complementary and alternative medicine (CAM) as a group of diverse medical and healthcare systems, practices, and products not generally considered part of conventional medicine.

Complementary medicine is used together with conventional medicine, and alternative medicine is used in place of conventional medicine. Integrative medicine combines conventional and CAM treatments for which there is evidence of safety and effectiveness. While scientific evidence exists regarding some CAM therapies, for most there are key questions that are yet to be answered through well-designed scientific studies questions such as whether these therapies are safe and whether they work for the purposes for which they are used. According to a report based on data from the National Health Interview Survey, nearly 12 percent of U.S. children and adolescents (aged 17 years and under) use some form of CAM.

Complementary And Alternative Medicine Information For Teens, Third Edition provides updated information about CAM systems, therapies, and practices, including various whole medical systems, manipulative practices, and movement therapies. Mind-body medicine, biologically based practices, energy medicine, and creative arts therapies are also discussed. A special section describes CAM therapies intended to help patients with specific diseases and conditions, such as cancer, diabetes, asthma, irritable bowel syndrome, and attention deficit hyperactivity disorder (ADHD). The book concludes with information about CAM clinical trials, suggestions for further reading, and a directory of CAM resources.

How To Use This Book

This book is divided into parts and chapters. Parts focus on broad areas of interest; chapters are devoted to single topics within a part.

Part One: Introduction To Complementary And Alternative Medicine defines CAM, provides statistics on CAM use in the United States, and describes how to evaluate web-based CAM information. It also includes suggestions for selecting a CAM practitioner.

Part Two: Whole Medical Systems explains systems of medicine that were built upon theories and practices that developed separately, and often independently, from the standard approach to medicine used among physicians in Western nations. These include traditional Chinese medicine, Ayurvedic medicine, homeopathy, and others.

Part Three: Manipulative Practices And Movement Therapies describes procedures based on the theory that different types of body repositioning can have an effect on health and well-being. Chiropractic medicine, kinesiotherapy, massage therapy, Rolfing structural integration, and Feldenkrais method are other techniques explained.

Part Four: Mind-Body Medicine discusses therapies that rely on focus and relaxation. These include biofeedback, meditation, hypnotherapy, aromatherapy, and guided imagery. Qi gong, tai chi, and yoga are also included, and spirituality as a form of CAM therapy is addressed.

Part Five: Biologically Based Practices provides facts about nutrition and health, dietary and antioxidant supplements, herbal medicine, and botanical products—including one of the most controversial: marijuana. It also explains biologically based practices, such as oral probiotics, enzyme therapy, and others. In addition, specialized diets (such as Fad diets and detoxification diets) are discussed.

Part Six: Energy Medicine describes practices purported to induce healing by manipulating the body's life force. These include acupuncture, which has been studied extensively related to its role in pain management and nausea relief, and others about which less is known, such as magnet therapy, therapeutic touch, and reiki.

Part Seven: Creative Arts Therapies discusses how art and music therapies can affect health in a positive way.

Part Eight: CAM Treatments For Cancer And Other Diseases And Conditions offers information about the types of complementary health therapies that are used most frequently for cancer, pain management, asthma, diabetes, irritable bowel syndrome, attention deficit hyperactivity disorder (ADHD), seasonal affective disorder (SAD), and other health concerns.

Part Nine: If You Need More Information includes facts about finding CAM clinical trials. It also provides suggestions for additional reading and a directory of organizations for further materials about CAM therapies and practices.

Bibliographic Note

This volume contains documents and excerpts from publications issued by the following government agencies: National Cancer Institute (NCI); National Center for

Complementary and Integrative Health (NCCIH); National Endowment For The Arts (NEA); National Institutes of Health (NIH); *News in Health*; Office of Dietary Supplements (ODS); Office of Disease Prevention and Health Promotion (ODPHP); Office of Family Assistance (OFA); Substance Abuse and Mental Health Services Administration (SAMHSA); U.S. Bureau of Labor Statistics (BLS); U.S. Department of Agriculture (USDA); U.S. Department of Education (ED); U.S. Department of Energy (DOE); U.S. Department of Health and Human Services (HHS); U.S. Department of Labor (DOL); U.S. Department of Veterans Affairs (VA); and U.S. Food and Drug Administration (FDA).

It may also contain original material produced by Omnigraphics and reviewed by medical consultants.

The photograph on the front cover is © wavebreakmedia.

Medical Review

Omnigraphics contracts with a team of qualified, senior medical professionals who serve as medical consultants for the *Teen Health Series*. As necessary, medical consultants review reprinted and originally written material for currency and accuracy. Citations including the phrase, Reviewed (month, year)" indicate material reviewed by this team. Medical consultation services are provided to the *Teen Health Series* editors by:

Dr. Vijayalakshmi, MBBS, DGO, MD
Dr. Senthil Selvan, MBBS, DCH, MD
Dr. K. Sivanandham, MBBS, DCH, MS (Research), PhD

About The *Teen Health Series*

At the request of librarians serving today's young adults, the *Teen Health Series* was developed as a specially focused set of volumes within Omnigraphics' *Health Reference Series*. Each volume deals comprehensively with a topic selected according to the needs and interests of people in middle school and high school. Teens seeking preventive guidance, information about disease warning signs, medical statistics, and risk factors for health problems will find answers to their questions in the *Teen Health Series*. The *Series*, however, is not intended to serve as a tool for diagnosing illness, in prescribing treatments, or as a substitute for the physician/patient relationship. All people concerned about medical symptoms or the possibility of disease are encouraged to seek professional care from an appropriate healthcare provider.

If there is a topic you would like to see addressed in a future volume of the *Teen Health Series*, please write to:

Editor
Teen Health Series
Omnigraphics
615 Griswold, Ste. 901
Detroit, MI 48226

A Note About Spelling And Style

Teen Health Series editors use *Stedman's Medical Dictionary* as an authority for questions related to the spelling of medical terms and the *Chicago Manual of Style* for questions related to grammatical structures, punctuation, and other editorial concerns. Consistent adherence is not always possible, however, because the individual volumes within the *Series* include many documents from a wide variety of different producers and copyright holders, and the editor's primary goal is to present material from each source as accurately as is possible following the terms specified by each document's producer. This sometimes means that information in different chapters may follow other guidelines and alternate spelling authorities. For example, occasionally a copyright holder may require that eponymous terms be shown in possessive forms (Crohn's disease vs. Crohn disease) or that British spelling norms be retained (leukaemia vs. leukemia).

Part One
Introduction To Complementary And Alternative Medicine

Chapter 1

What Is Complementary And Alternative Medicine (CAM)?

Complementary and alternative medicine (CAM) is the term for medical products and practices that are not part of standard medical care.

- **Standard medical care** is medicine that is practiced by health professionals who hold an M.D. (medical doctor) or D.O. (doctor of osteopathy) degree. It is also practiced by other health professionals, such as physical therapists, physician assistants, psychologists, and registered nurses. Standard medicine may also be called biomedicine or allopathic, Western, mainstream, orthodox, or regular medicine. Some standard medical care practitioners are also practitioners of CAM.
- **Complementary medicine** is treatments that are used along with standard medical treatments but are not considered to be standard treatments. One example is using acupuncture to help lessen some side effects of cancer treatment.
- **Alternative medicine** is treatments that are used instead of standard medical treatments. One example is using a special diet to treat cancer instead of anticancer drugs that are prescribed by an oncologist.
- **Integrative medicine** is a total approach to medical care that combines standard medicine with the CAM practices that have been shown to be safe and effective. They treat the patient's mind, body, and spirit.

About This Chapter: Text in this chapter begins with excerpts from "Complementary And Alternative Medicine," National Cancer Institute (NCI), April 10, 2015; Text beginning with the heading "Integrative Medicine" is excerpted from "Complementary, Alternative, Or Integrative Health: What's In A Name?" National Center for Complementary and Integrative Health (NCCIH), June 2016.

Complementary means using a nonmainstream practice together with conventional medicine. Alternative means using nonmainstream practices in place of conventional medicine. For instance, using an herb to manage your *multiple sclerosis* (*MS*) alone would be alternative. Using an herb together with an MS disease-modifying drug would be complementary. Bringing conventional and complementary approaches together in a coordinated way is known as "integrative" healthcare.

(Source: "Complementary And Alternative Medicine And Whole Health," U.S. Department of Veterans Affairs (VA).)

Are CAM Approaches Safe?

Some CAM therapies have undergone careful evaluation and have been found to be safe and effective. However there are others that have been found to be ineffective or possibly harmful. Less is known about many CAM therapies, and research has been slower for a number of reasons:

- Time and funding issues
- Problems finding institutions and cancer researchers to work with on the studies
- Regulatory issues

CAM therapies need to be evaluated with the same long and careful research process used to evaluate standard treatments. Standard cancer treatments have generally been studied for safety and effectiveness through an intense scientific process that includes clinical trials with large numbers of patients.

Natural Does Not Mean Safe

CAM therapies include a wide variety of botanicals and nutritional products, such as dietary supplements, herbal supplements, and vitamins. Many of these "natural" products are considered to be safe because they are present in, or produced by, nature. However, that is not true in all cases. In addition, some may affect how well other medicines work in your body. For example, the herb St. John's wort, which some people use for depression, may cause certain anticancer drugs not to work as well as they should.

Herbal supplements may be harmful when taken by themselves, with other substances, or in large doses. For example, some studies have shown that kava kava, an herb that has been used to help with stress and anxiety, may cause liver damage.

Vitamins can also have unwanted effects in your body. For example, some studies show that high doses of vitamins, even vitamin C, may affect how chemotherapy and radiation work. Too much of any vitamin is not safe, even in a healthy person.

Tell your doctor if you're taking any dietary supplements, no matter how safe you think they are. This is very important. Even though there may be ads or claims that something has been used for years, they do not prove that it's safe or effective.

Supplements do not have to be approved by the federal government before being sold to the public. Also, a prescription is not needed to buy them. Therefore, it's up to consumers to decide what is best for them.

What Should Patients Do When Using Or Considering CAM Therapies?

Patients who are using or considering using complementary or alternative therapy should talk with their doctor or nurse. Some therapies may interfere with standard treatment or even be harmful. It is also a good idea to learn whether the therapy has been proven to do what it claims to do.

To find a CAM practitioner, ask your doctor or nurse to suggest someone. Or ask if someone at your healthcare center, such as a social worker or physical therapist can help you. Choosing a CAM practitioner should be done with as much care as choosing a primary care provider.

Integrative Medicine

There are many definitions of "integrative" healthcare, but all involve bringing conventional and complementary approaches together in a coordinated way. The use of integrative approaches to health and wellness has grown within care settings across the United States. Researchers are exploring the potential benefits of integrative health in a variety of situations, including pain management for military personnel and veterans, relief of symptoms in cancer patients and survivors, and programs to promote healthy behaviors.

Integrative Approaches And Health-Related Behaviors

Healthy behaviors, such as eating right, getting enough physical activity, and not smoking, can reduce people's risks of developing serious diseases. Can integrative approaches promote these types of behaviors? Researchers are working to answer this question. Preliminary research suggests that yoga and meditation-based therapies may help smokers quit, and National Center for Complementary and Integrative Health (NCCIH)-funded studies are testing whether adding mindfulness-based approaches to weight control programs will help people lose weight more successfully.

Types Of Complementary Health Approaches

Most complementary health approaches fall into one of two subgroups—natural products or mind and body practices.

Natural Products

This group includes a variety of products, such as herbs (also known as botanicals), vitamins and minerals, and probiotics. They are widely marketed, readily available to consumers, and often sold as dietary supplements.

According to the 2012 National Health Interview Survey (NHIS), which included a comprehensive survey on the use of complementary health approaches by Americans, 17.7 percent of American adults had used a dietary supplement other than vitamins and minerals in the past year. These products were the most popular complementary health approach in the survey. The most commonly used natural product was fish oil.

Researchers have done large, rigorous studies on a few natural products, but the results often showed that the products didn't work. Research on others is in progress. While there are indications that some may be helpful, more needs to be learned about the effects of these products in the human body and about their safety and potential interactions with medicines and other natural products.

Mind And Body Practices

Mind and body practices include a large and diverse group of procedures or techniques administered or taught by a trained practitioner or teacher. The 2012 National Health Insurance Scheme (NHIS) showed that yoga, chiropractic and osteopathic manipulation, meditation, and massage therapy are among the most popular mind and body practices used by adults. The popularity of yoga has grown dramatically in recent years, with almost twice as many U.S. adults practicing yoga in 2012 as in 2002.

Other mind and body practices include acupuncture, relaxation techniques (such as breathing exercises, guided imagery, and progressive muscle relaxation), tai chi, qi gong, healing touch, hypnotherapy, and movement therapies (such as Feldenkrais method, Alexander technique, Pilates, Rolfing structural integration, and Trager psychophysical integration).

The amount of research on mind and body approaches varies widely depending on the practice. For example, researchers have done many studies on acupuncture, yoga, spinal manipulation, and meditation, but there have been fewer studies on some other practices.

> Nearly 12 percent of children and teens (about one in nine) in the United States are using some form of complementary health product or practice, such as chiropractic or spinal manipulation, yoga, meditation, or massage therapy.
>
> *(Source: "7 Things To Know About Mind And Body Practices For Children And Teens," National Center for Complementary and Integrative Health (NCCIH).)*

Other Complementary Health Approaches

The two broad areas discussed above—natural products and mind and body practices—capture most complementary health approaches. However, some approaches may not neatly fit into either of these groups—for example, the practices of traditional healers, Ayurvedic medicine, traditional Chinese medicine, homeopathy, and naturopathy.

Chapter 2

Use Of CAM In The United States

In the past, children were often excluded from research studies due to special protections, and findings from studies of adults were applied to children. Today, the National Institutes of Health (NIH) requires that children be included in all studies, unless there are scientific and ethical reasons not to.

Patterns In The Use Of Complementary Health Approaches For Children

The National Health Interview Survey (NHIS) included a comprehensive survey on the use of complementary health approaches by almost 45,000 Americans, including more than 10,000 children aged 4–17. The survey found that 11.6 percent of the children had used or been given some form of complementary health product or practice, such as yoga or dietary supplements, during the past year.

The most frequently used approaches for children were natural products (fish oil, melatonin, and probiotics), and chiropractic or osteopathic manipulation.

For children, complementary health approaches were most often used for back or neck pain, other musculoskeletal conditions, head or chest colds, anxiety or stress, attention deficit hyperactivity disorder (ADHD) or attention deficit disorder (ADD), and insomnia or trouble sleeping.

About This Chapter: This chapter includes text excerpted from "Children And The Use Of Complementary Health Approaches," National Center for Complementary and Integrative Health (NCCIH), March 2017.

Other studies show that children in the United States who use or are given complementary health approaches vary in age and health status. For example:

- Teens are particularly likely to use products that claim to improve sports performance, increase energy levels, or promote weight loss.
- Children with chronic medical conditions, including anxiety, musculoskeletal conditions, and recurrent headaches, are more likely than other children to use complementary health approaches, usually along with conventional care.

What The Science Says About The Safety And Side Effects Of Complementary Health Approaches For Children

- Dietary supplements result in about 23,000 emergency room visits every year. Many of the patients are young adults who come to the emergency room with heart problems from taking weight-loss or energy products. One-fifth of the visits are children; most of whom took a vitamin or mineral when unsupervised. (Child-resistant packaging isn't required for dietary supplements.)
- Some dietary supplements contain contaminants, including drugs, chemicals, or metals.
- Children's small size, developing organs, and immature immune system make them more vulnerable than adults to having allergic or other adverse reactions to dietary supplements.
- Some products may worsen conditions. For example, echinacea is a type of ragweed so people sensitive to ragweed may also react to echinacea.
- Do not rely on asthma products sold over-the-counter (OTC) and labeled as homeopathic, the U.S. Food and Drug Administration (FDA) warns. Homeopathic remedies and dietary supplements are not evaluated by the FDA for safety or effectiveness.
- Biofeedback, guided imagery, hypnosis, mindfulness, and yoga are some of the mind and body practices that have the best evidence of being effective for children for various symptoms (such as anxiety and stress) and are low-risk. However, spinal manipulation, a common complementary approach, is associated with rare but serious complications.

More To Consider

- Make sure that you have received an accurate diagnosis from a licensed healthcare provider.

- Educate yourself about the potential risks and benefits of complementary health approaches.
    - Ask your healthcare provider about the effectiveness and possible risks of approaches you're considering or already using for yourself.
- Do not replace or delay conventional care or prescribed medications with any health product or practice that hasn't been proven safe and effective.
- If a healthcare provider suggests a complementary approach, do not increase the dose or duration of the treatment beyond what is recommended (more isn't necessarily better).
- If you have any concerns about the effects of a complementary approach, contact your healthcare provider.
- As with all medications and other potentially harmful products, store dietary supplements out of the sight and reach of children.
- The National Center for Complementary and Integrative Health (NCCIH) website offers safety tips on dietary supplements and mind and body practices for children and teens.
- Tell all your healthcare providers about any complementary or integrative health approaches you use. Give them a full picture of what you do to manage your health. This will help ensure coordinated and safe care.

Selecting A Complementary Health Practitioner

If you're looking for a complementary health practitioner for yourself, be as careful and thorough in your search as you are when looking for conventional care. Be sure to ask about the practitioner's:

- Experience in coordinating care with conventional healthcare providers.
- Experience in delivering care to children and adolescents.
- Education, training, and license.

Chapter 3

Are You Considering Complementary Medicine?

Millions of Americans use complementary health approaches. Like any decision concerning your health, decisions about whether to use complementary approaches are important. This chapter will assist you in your decision making about complementary health products and practices.

What Do "Complementary," "Alternative," And "Integrative" Mean?

"Complementary and alternative medicine," "complementary medicine," "alternative medicine," "integrative medicine"—you may have seen these terms on the Internet and in marketing, but what do they really mean? While the terms are often used to mean the array of healthcare approaches with a history of use or origins outside of mainstream medicine, they are actually hard to define and may mean different things to different people.

The terms complementary and integrative refer to the use of nonmainstream approaches together with conventional medical approaches.

Alternative health approaches refer to the use of nonmainstream products or practices in place of conventional medicine. National Center for Complementary and Integrative Health (NCCIH) advises against using any product or practice that has not been proven safe and effective as a substitute for conventional medical treatment or as a reason

About This Chapter: This chapter includes text excerpted from "Are You Considering A Complementary Health Approach?" National Center for Complementary and Integrative Health (NCCIH), September 2016.

to postpone seeing your healthcare provider about any health problem. In some instances, stopping—or not starting—conventional treatment can have serious consequences. Before making a decision not to use a proven conventional treatment, talk to your healthcare providers.

How Can I Get Reliable Information About A Complementary Health Approach?

It's important to learn what scientific studies have discovered about the complementary health approach you're considering. Evidence from research studies is stronger and more reliable than something you've seen in an advertisement or on a website, or something someone told you about that worked for them.

Understanding a product's or practice's potential benefits, risks, and scientific evidence is critical to your health and safety. Scientific research on many complementary health approaches is relatively new, so this kind of information may not be available for each one. However, many studies are under way, including those that NCCIH supports, and knowledge and understanding of complementary approaches are increasing all the time. Here are some ways to find reliable information:

- **Talk with your healthcare providers.** Tell them about the complementary health approach you're considering and ask any questions you may have about safety, effectiveness, or interactions with medications (prescription or nonprescription) or dietary supplements.
- **Visit the NCCIH website (nccih.nih.gov).** The "Health Information" page has an A–Z list of complementary health products and practices, which describes what the science says about them, and links to other objective sources of online information. The website also has contact information for the NCCIH Clearinghouse, where information specialists are available to assist you in searching the scientific literature and to suggest useful NCCIH publications. You can also find information from NCCIH on Facebook (www.facebook.com/nih.nccih), Twitter (www.twitter.com/nih_nccih), YouTube (www.youtube.com/c/nih_nccih), and Pinterest (www.pinterest.com/nccih).
- **Visit your local library or a medical library.** Ask the reference librarian to help you find scientific journals and trustworthy books with information on the product or practice that interests you.

Be An Informed Consumer

Decisions about your healthcare are important—including decisions about whether or not to use complementary health products and practices. Take charge of your health by being an informed consumer. Find out and consider what scientific studies have been done on the safety and effectiveness of the product or practice that interests you. Discuss the information with your healthcare provider before making a decision.

(Source: "Be An Informed Consumer," National Center for Complementary and Integrative Health (NCCIH).)

Are Complementary Health Approaches Safe?

As with any medical product or treatment, there can be risks with complementary approaches. These risks depend on the specific product or practice. Each needs to be considered on its own. However, if you're considering a specific product or practice, the following general suggestions can help you think about safety and minimize risks.

- Be aware that individuals respond differently to health products and practices, whether conventional or complementary. How you might respond to one depends on many things, including your state of health, how you use it, or your belief in it.
- Keep in mind that "natural" does not necessarily mean "safe." (Think of mushrooms that grow in the wild: some are safe to eat, while others are not.)
- Learn about factors that affect safety. For a practice that is administered by a practitioner, such as chiropractic, these factors include the training, skill, and experience of the practitioner. For a product such as a dietary supplement, the specific ingredients and the quality of the manufacturing process are important factors.
- If you decide to use a practice provided by a complementary health practitioner, choose the practitioner as carefully as you would your primary healthcare provider. If you decide to use a dietary supplement, such as an herbal product, be aware that some products may interact in harmful ways with medications (prescription or over the-counter (OTC)) or other dietary supplements, and some may have side effects on their own.
- Tell all your healthcare providers about any complementary or integrative health approaches you use. Give them a full picture of what you do to manage your health. This will help ensure coordinated and safe care.

To minimize the health risks of a nonmainstream treatment:

- Discuss it with your doctor. It might have side effects or interact with other medicines.
- Find out what the research says about it
- Choose practitioners carefully
- Tell all of your doctors and practitioners about all of the different types of treatments you use

(Source: "Complementary And Integrative Medicine," MedlinePlus, National Institutes of Health (NIH).)

How Can I Determine Whether Statements Made About The Effectiveness Of A Complementary Health Approach Are True?

Before you begin using a complementary health approach, it's a good idea to ask the following questions:

- Is there scientific evidence (not just personal stories) to backup the statements?
- What is the source? Statements that manufacturers or other promoters of some complementary health approaches may make about effectiveness and benefits can sound reasonable and promising. However, the statements may be based on a biased view of the available scientific evidence.
- How does the provider or manufacturer describe the approach?
    - Beware of terms like "scientific breakthrough," "miracle cure," "secret ingredient," or "ancient remedy."
    - If you encounter claims of a "quick fix" that depart from previous research, keep in mind that science usually advances over time by small steps, slowly building an evidence base.
    - Remember: if it sounds too good to be true—for example, claims that a product or practice can cure a disease or works for a variety of ailments—it usually is.

Are Complementary Health Approaches Tested To See If They Work?

While scientific evidence now exists regarding the effectiveness and safety of some complementary health approaches, there remain many yet to be answered questions about whether others are safe, whether they work for the diseases or medical conditions for which they are promoted, and how those approaches with health benefits may work. As the Federal Government's lead agency for scientific research on health interventions, practices, products, and disciplines that originate from outside mainstream medicine, NCCIH supports scientific research to answer these questions and determine who might benefit most from the use of specific approaches.

I'm Interested In An Approach That Involves Seeing A Complementary Health Practitioner. How Do I Go About Selecting A Practitioner?

- Your primary healthcare provider or local hospital may be able to recommend a complementary health practitioner.
- The professional organization for the type of practitioner you're seeking may have helpful information, such as licensing and training requirements. Many states have regulatory agencies or licensing boards for certain types of complementary health practitioners; they may be able to help you locate practitioners in your area.
- Make sure any practitioner you're considering is willing to work in collaboration with your other healthcare providers.

Chapter 4

Tell Your Healthcare Provider About Your CAM Use

When patients tell their providers about their use of complementary health practices, they can better stay in control and more effectively manage their health. When providers ask their patients, they can ensure that they are fully informed and can help patients make wise healthcare decisions.

Using CAM: Talk To Your Healthcare Provider

In an era of genomics and personalized medicine, we need to remember that a key ingredient to good healthcare is the dialogue you, as a patient, have with your providers. Talking not only allows integrated care, it also minimizes risks of interactions with a patient's conventional treatments. When patients tell their providers about their CAM use, they can more effectively manage their health. When providers ask their patients about CAM use, they can ensure that they are fully informed and can help patients make wise healthcare decisions.

(Source: "Time To Talk About CAM: Health Care Providers And Patients Need To Ask And Tell," National Center for Complementary and Integrative Health (NCCIH).)

Here are four tips to help you and your healthcare providers start talking:

1. **List the complementary health practices you use on your patient history form.** When completing the patient history form, be sure to include everything you

---

About This Chapter: Text in this chapter begins with excerpts from "4 Tips: Start Talking With Your Healthcare Providers About Complementary Health Approaches," National Center for Complementary and Integrative Health (NCCIH), September 24, 2017; Text under the heading "Patient Tips For Discussing CAM With Providers" is excerpted from "Time To Talk About CAM: Health Care Providers And Patients Need To Ask And Tell," National Center for Complementary and Integrative Health (NCCIH), June 4, 2015.

use—from acupuncture to zinc. It's important to give healthcare providers a full picture of what you do to manage your health.

2. **At each visit, be sure to tell your providers about what complementary health approaches you are using.** Don't forget to include over-the-counter (OTC) and prescription medicines, as well as dietary and herbal supplements. Make a list in advance and take it with you. Some complementary health approaches can have an effect on conventional medicine, so your provider needs to know.
3. **If you are considering a new complementary health practice, ask questions.** Ask your healthcare providers about its safety, effectiveness, and possible interactions with medications (both prescription and nonprescription).
4. **Don't wait for your providers to ask about any complementary health practice you are using.** Be proactive. Start the conversation.

Patient Tips For Discussing CAM With Providers

- When completing patient history forms, be sure to include all therapies and treatments you use. Make a list in advance.
- Tell your healthcare providers about all therapies or treatments including over-the-counter and prescription medicines, as well as dietary and herbal supplements.
- Take control. Don't wait for your providers to ask about your CAM use.
- If you are considering a new CAM therapy, ask your healthcare providers about its safety, effectiveness, and possible interactions with medicines (both prescription and over-the-counter).

Provider Tips For Discussing CAM With Patients

- Include a question about CAM use on medical history forms.
- Ask your patients to bring a list of all therapies they use, including prescription, over-the-counter, herbal therapies, and other CAM practices.
- Have your medical staff initiate the conversation.

(Source: "Time To Talk About CAM: Health Care Providers And Patients Need To Ask And Tell," National Center for Complementary and Integrative Health (NCCIH).)

Chapter 5

Evaluating Web-Based Health Resources

The number of websites offering health related resources—including information about complementary health approaches (often called complementary and alternative medicine)—grows every day. Social media sites have also become an important source of online health information for some people. Many online health resources are useful, but others may present information that is inaccurate or misleading, so it's important to find sources you can trust and to know how to evaluate their content. This chapter provides help for finding reliable websites and outlines things to consider in evaluating health information from websites and social media sources.

Checking Out A Health Website: Five Quick Questions

If you're visiting a health website for the first time, these five quick questions can help you decide whether the site is a helpful resource.

Who? Who runs the website? Can you trust them?

What? What does the site say? Do its claims seem too good to be true?

When? When was the information posted or reviewed? Is it up-to-date?

Where? Where did the information come from? Is it based on scientific research?

Why? Why does the site exist? Is it selling something?

About This Chapter: This chapter includes text excerpted from "Finding And Evaluating Online Resources," National Center for Complementary and Integrative Health (NCCIH), September 2014. Reviewed January 2018.

Who Runs And Pays For The Website?

Any reliable health related website should make it easy for you to learn who's responsible for the site. For example, on the National Center for Complementary and Integrative Health (NCCIH) website, each major page clearly identifies NCCIH and, because NCCIH is part of NIH, provides a link to the NIH homepage. If it isn't obvious who runs the website, look for a link on the homepage to an "About This Site" page.

You can also learn about who runs a website by looking at the letters at the end of its Web address. For example, Web addresses (such as NCCIH's) that end in ".gov" mean it's a government-sponsored site; ".edu" indicates an educational institution, ".org" a noncommercial organization, and ".com" a commercial organization.

You can trust sites with ".gov" addresses. You can also trust sites with ".edu" addresses if they're produced by the educational institution. Personal pages of individuals at an educational institution may not be trustworthy, even though they have ".edu" addresses. The presence of ".org" in an address doesn't guarantee that a site is reputable; there have been instances where phony ".org" sites were set up to mislead consumers. Also, some legitimate ".org" sites belong to organizations that promote a specific agenda; their content may be biased.

You should know how the site supports itself. Is it funded by the organization that sponsors it? Does it sell advertising? Is it sponsored by a company that sells dietary supplements, drugs, or other products or services? The source of funding can affect what content is presented, how it's presented, and what the site owners want to accomplish.

What Is The Purpose Of The Site?

The site's purpose is related to who runs and pays for it. The About This Site page should include a clear statement of purpose. To be sure you're getting reliable information, you should confirm information that you find on sales sites by consulting other, independent sites where no products are sold.

What Is The Source Of The Information?

Many health/medical sites post information collected from other websites or sources. If the person or organization in charge of the site didn't create the material, the original source should be clearly identified. For example, the Health Topics A–Z page on the NCCIH site provides links to some documents that NCCIH didn't create; in those instances, the source of the documents is always identified.

What Is The Basis Of The Information?

In addition to identifying the source of the material you're reading, the site should describe the evidence (such as articles in medical journals) that the material is based on. Also, opinions or advice should be clearly set apart from information that's "evidence-based" (that is, based on research results). For example, if a site discusses health benefits people can expect from a treatment, look for references to scientific research that clearly support what's said. Keep in mind that testimonials, anecdotes, unsupported claims, and opinions aren't the same as objective, evidence-based information.

Is The Information Reviewed?

You can be more confident in the quality of medical information on a website if people with credible professional and scientific qualifications review the material before it's posted. Some websites have an editorial board that reviews content. Others put the names and credentials of the individuals who reviewed a webpage in an Acknowledgments section near the end of the page.

How Current Is The Information?

Some types of outdated medical information can be misleading or even dangerous. Responsible health websites review and update much of their content on a regular basis, especially informational content such as fact sheets and lists of frequently asked questions (FAQs). Other types of site content, however, such as news reports or summaries of scientific meetings, may never be updated; their purpose is to describe an event, rather than to provide the most up-to-date information on a topic.

What Is The Site's Policy About Linking To Other Sites?

Websites usually have a policy about establishing links to other sites. Some sites take a conservative approach and don't link to any other sites. Some link to any site that asks or pays for a link. Others only link to sites that have met certain criteria. You may be able to find information on the site about its linking policy. (For example, you can find information about NCCIH's linking policy on the NCCIH website Information and Policies page at www.nccih.nih.gov/tools/privacy.htm.) Unless the site's linking policy is strict, don't assume that the sites that it links to are reliable. You should evaluate the linked sites just as you would any other site that you're visiting for the first time.

How Does The Site Handle Personal Information?

Many websites track visitors' paths to determine what pages are being viewed. A health website may ask you to "subscribe" or "become a member." In some cases, this may be so that it can collect a user fee or select information for you that's relevant to your concerns. In all cases, this will give the site personal information about you.

Any credible site asking for this kind of information should tell you exactly what it will and will not do with it. Many commercial sites sell "aggregate" (collected) data about their users to other companies—information such as what percentage of their users are women older than 40. In some cases, they may collect and reuse information that's "personally identifiable," such as your ZIP Code, gender, and birth date. Be sure to read any privacy policy or similar language on the site, and don't sign up for anything you don't fully understand. You can find NCCIH's privacy policy at www.nccih.nih.gov/tools/privacy.htm#privacy.

How To Protect Yourself

If you suspect that a news site is fake, look for a disclaimer somewhere on the page (often in small print) that indicates that the site is an advertisement. Also, don't rely on Internet news reports when making important decisions about your health. If you're considering a health product described in the news, discuss it with your healthcare provider.

How Does The Site Manage Interactions With Users?

You should always be able to contact the site owner if you run across problems or have questions or feedback. If the site hosts online discussion areas (forums or message boards), it should explain the terms of using this service. If the site is affiliated with social networking sites such as Twitter, Facebook, or YouTube, it should explain the terms of using them. Look for a social media comments policy on the website. NCCIH's social media comments policy is here: www.nccih.nih.gov/tools/commentpolicy.htm. Spend some time reading what has been posted before joining in to see whether you feel comfortable with the environment. You may also be able to review past discussions.

Chapter 6

Selecting A CAM Practitioner

If you're looking for a complementary health practitioner to help treat a medical problem, it is important to be as careful and thorough in your search as you are when looking for conventional care.

Here are some tips to help you in your search:

- **If you need names of practitioners in your area, first check with your doctor or other healthcare provider.** A nearby hospital or medical school, professional organizations, state regulatory agencies or licensing boards, or even your health insurance provider may be helpful. Unfortunately, the National Center for Complementary and Integrative Health (NCCIH) cannot refer you to practitioners.
- **Find out as much as you can about any potential practitioner, including education, training, licensing, and certifications.** The credentials required for complementary health practitioners vary tremendously from state to state and from discipline to discipline.

Once you have found a possible practitioner, here are some tips about deciding whether he or she is right for you:

- **Find out whether the practitioner is willing to work together with your conventional healthcare providers.** For safe, coordinated care, it's important for all of the professionals involved in your health to communicate and cooperate.

About This Chapter: Text in this chapter begins with excerpts from "6 Things To Know When Selecting A Complementary Health Practitioner," National Center for Complementary and Integrative Health (NCCIH), September 24, 2017; Text beginning with the heading "Credentialing, Licensing, Certifying—What's The Difference?" is excerpted from "Credentialing, Licensing, And Education," National Center for Complementary and Integrative Health (NCCIH), October 2015.

- **Explain all of your health conditions to the practitioner, and find out about the practitioner's training and experience in working with people who have your conditions.** Choose a practitioner who understands how to work with people with your specific needs, even if general well-being is your goal. And, remember that health conditions can affect the safety of complementary approaches; for example, if you have glaucoma, some yoga poses may not be safe for you.
- **Don't assume that your health insurance will cover the practitioner's services.** Contact your health insurance provider and ask. Insurance plans differ greatly in what complementary health approaches they cover, and even if they cover a particular approach, restrictions may apply.
- **Tell all your healthcare providers about the complementary approaches you use and about all practitioners who are treating you.** Keeping your healthcare providers fully informed helps you to stay in control and effectively manage your health.

Credentialing, Licensing, Certifying—What's The Difference?

Credentials is a broad term that can refer to a practitioner's license, certification, or education. Government agencies grant and monitor licenses; professional organizations certify practitioners.

Certification can be either a prerequisite for licensure or, in some cases, an alternative. To get certified or licensed, practitioners must meet specific education, training, or practice standards. Being licensed or certified is not a guarantee of being qualified.

States use the following approaches to credential practitioners:

- **Mandatory licensure:** requires practitioners to have a license for providing a service.
- **Title licensure:** requires practitioners to have credentials before using a professional title.
- **Registration:** requires practitioners to provide information about their training and experience to a state consumer protection agency.

States' requirements for granting a license vary considerably. They may require those seeking a license to do one or more of the following:

- Graduate from a certified program.
- Meet certification requirements of a national organization.

- Complete a specified amount of training.
- Pass a written exam (sometimes a practical exam is also required).
- Participate in continuing education.

States also vary widely in the services that they allow complementary health practitioners to offer patients. For example, some states permit acupuncturists to recommend dietary supplements to their patients, while other states specifically prohibit it.

Education And Training

Professional organizations offer certification examinations to graduates of accredited education and training programs. Certification qualifies them for state or local licensure. For example, in many states acupuncturists who do not have a doctor of medicine (M.D.) degree must be certified by the National Certification Commission for Acupuncture and Oriental Medicine (NCCAOM) to get licensed. Some of the other professional organizations involved in certification include the National Certification Board for Therapeutic Massage & Bodywork (NCBTMB), the Council for Homeopathic Certification (CHC), the National Board of Chiropractic Examiners (NBCE), and the North American Board of Naturopathic Examiners (NABNE).

Schools and educational programs across the country train complementary health practitioners and prepare them for certification in their field. The U.S. Department of Education (ED) authorizes specific organizations to accredit education or training programs. For example, it has authorized the Council on Chiropractic Education (CCE) to accredit chiropractic colleges and the Accreditation Commission for Acupuncture and Oriental Medicine (ACAOM) to accredit acupuncture programs.

Chapter 7

Paying For Complementary And Integrative Health Approaches

Use Of Complementary Health Approaches In The United States

Data from the 2012 National Health Interview Survey (NHIS) show that 33 percent of adults and almost 12 percent of children use complementary health approaches, and that the most commonly used approach is natural products (dietary supplements other than vitamins and minerals). Fish oil is the natural product most often used by adults and children. As for mind and body practices, adults and children most often turn to chiropractic or osteopathic manipulation, yoga, meditation, and massage therapy.

Out-Of-Pocket Spending On Complementary Health Approaches

People seem to be willing to pay "out-of-pocket" (not through insurance) for certain complementary health approaches. In fact, out-of-pocket spending on these approaches for Americans age 4 and older amounts to an estimated $30.2 billion per year, according to the 2012 NHIS. This includes:

- $14.7 billion out-of-pocket for visits to complementary and integrative health practitioners such as chiropractors, acupuncturists, and massage therapists
- $12.8 billion out-of-pocket on natural products

About This Chapter: This chapter includes text excerpted from "Paying For Complementary And Integrative Health Approaches," National Center for Complementary and Integrative Health (NCCIH), June 2016.

- About $2.7 billion on self-care approaches (homeopathic medicines and self-help materials, such as books or CDs, related to complementary health topics).
- This out-of-pocket spending for complementary health approaches represents 9.2 percent of all out-of-pocket spending by Americans on healthcare ($328.8 billion) and 1.1 percent of total healthcare spending ($2.82 trillion).

Insurance Coverage Of Complementary Health Approaches

Many Americans use complementary health approaches, but the type of health insurance they have affects their decisions to use these practices. In a 2012 study, researchers analyzed NHIS data on acupuncture, chiropractic, and massage—and compared that with data from 2002. While use rates for all three approaches rose, the increase was much more pronounced among those who did not have health insurance. For those who had health insurance, coverage for these three approaches was more likely to be partial than full.

If you would like to use a complementary or integrative approach and don't know if your health insurance will cover it, you should contact your health insurance provider to find out.

Some questions to ask your insurance provider include:

- Is this complementary or integrative approach covered for my health condition?
- Does it need to be
- Preauthorized or preapproved?
- Ordered by a prescription?
- Do I need a referral?
- Does coverage require seeing a practitioner in the network?
- Do I have coverage if I go out-of-network?
- Are there any limits and requirements—for example, on the number of visits or the amount you will pay?
- How much do I have to pay out-of-pocket?

Keep records about all contacts you have with your insurance company, including notes on calls and copies of bills, claims, and letters. This may help if you have a claim dispute.

If you're choosing a new health insurance plan, ask the insurance provider about coverage of complementary or integrative health approaches. You should find out if you need a special "rider" or supplement to the standard plan for these approaches to be covered. You should also find out if the insurer offers a discount program in which plan members pay for fees and products out-of-pocket but at a lower rate.

General information on health plans and benefits is available from the U.S. Department of Labor (DOL).

Sources Of Information On Insurers

Your state insurance department may be able to help you determine which insurance companies cover specific complementary or integrative health approaches. USA.gov provides contact information for state and local consumer agencies, including insurance regulators.

Professional associations for complementary health specialties may monitor insurance coverage and reimbursement in their field. You can ask a reference librarian for help or search for them on the Internet.

Asking Practitioners About Payment

If you're planning to see a complementary or integrative practitioner, it's important to understand about payment. Here are some questions to ask:

- Costs: What does the first appointment cost? What do followup appointments cost? Is there a sliding scale based on income? How many appointments am I likely to need? Are there other costs (e.g., tests, equipment, supplements)?
- Insurance: Do you accept my insurance plan? What has been your experience with my plan's coverage for people with my condition? Do I file the claims, or do you take care of that?

Federal Health Benefit Programs

The Federal Government helps with some health expenses of people who are eligible for Federal health benefit programs, such as programs for veterans, people aged 65 and older (Medicare), and people who cannot afford healthcare (Medicaid, funded jointly with the states).

Information on health benefits for veterans is available from the U.S. Department of Veterans Affairs (VA). Information on Medicare and Medicaid is available from the Centers for Medicare and Medicaid Services. A handbook, *Medicare* & *You*, explains what services Medicare covers.

Two other Internet resources—Benefits.gov and the Health and Insurance page on the OPM website—explain Federal health benefit programs. Benefits.gov has a benefits-finder that can help you learn more about qualifying for programs.

Part Two
Whole Medical Systems

Chapter 8

Understanding Whole Medical Systems

Whole medical systems involve complete systems of theory and practice that have evolved independently from or parallel to allopathic (conventional) medicine. Many are traditional systems of medicine that are practiced by individual cultures throughout the world. Major Eastern whole medical systems include traditional Chinese medicine (TCM) and Ayurvedic medicine, one of India's traditional systems of medicine. Major Western whole medical systems include homeopathy and naturopathy. Other systems have been developed by Native American, African, Middle Eastern, Tibetan, and Central and South American cultures.

Traditional Chinese Medicine (TCM)

TCM is a complete system of healing that dates back to 200 B.C. in written form. Korea, Japan, and Vietnam have all developed their own unique versions of traditional medicine based on practices originating in China. In the TCM view, the body is a delicate balance of two opposing and inseparable forces: yin and yang. Yin represents the cold, slow, or passive principle, while yang represents the hot, excited, or active principle. Among the major assumptions in TCM are that health is achieved by maintaining the body in a "balanced state" and that disease is due to an internal imbalance of yin and yang. This imbalance leads to blockage in the flow of qi (or vital energy) and of blood along pathways known as meridians. TCM

About This Chapter: Text in this chapter begins with excerpts from "Whole Medical Systems: An Overview," National Center for Complementary and Integrative Health (NCCIH), October 2004. Reviewed January 2018; Text under the heading "Native American Medicine" is excerpted from "Healing Ways," U.S. National Library of Medicine (NLM), September 26, 2011. Reviewed January 2018.

practitioners typically use herbs, acupuncture, and massage to help unblock qi and blood in patients in an attempt to bring the body back into harmony and wellness.

Treatments in TCM are typically tailored to the subtle patterns of disharmony in each patient and are based on an individualized diagnosis. The diagnostic tools differ from those of conventional medicine. There are three main therapeutic modalities:

1. Acupuncture and moxibustion (moxibustion is the application of heat from the burning of the herb moxa at the acupuncture point)
2. Chinese *Materia Medica* (the catalogue of natural products used in TCM)
3. Massage and manipulation

Although TCM proposes that natural products catalogued in Chinese *Materia Medica* or acupuncture can be used alone to treat virtually any illness, quite often they are used together and sometimes in combination with other modalities (e.g., massage, moxibustion, diet changes, or exercise).

What Is Traditional Chinese Medicine (TCM)?

A medical system that has been used for thousands of years to prevent, diagnose, and treat disease. It is based on the belief that qi (the body's vital energy) flows along meridians (channels) in the body and keeps a person's spiritual, emotional, mental, and physical health in balance. Traditional Chinese medicine aims to restore the body's balance and harmony between the natural opposing forces of yin and yang, which can block qi and cause disease. Traditional Chinese medicine includes acupuncture, diet, herbal therapy, meditation, physical exercise, and massage. Also called Oriental medicine.

(Source: "NCI Dictionary Of Cancer Terms," National Cancer Institute (NCI).)

Acupuncture

A report from a Consensus Development Conference on Acupuncture held at the National Institutes of Health (NIH) states that acupuncture is being "widely" practiced—by thousands of acupuncturists, physicians, dentists, and other practitioners—for relief or prevention of pain and for various other health conditions. In terms of the evidence at that time, acupuncture was considered to have potential clinical value for nausea/vomiting and dental pain, and limited evidence suggested its potential in the treatment of other pain disorders, paralysis and numbness, movement disorders, depression, insomnia, breathlessness, and asthma.

Preclinical studies have documented acupuncture's effects, but they have not been able to fully explain how acupuncture works within the framework of the Western system of medicine.

It is proposed that acupuncture produces its effects by the conduction of electromagnetic signals at a greater-than-normal rate, thus aiding the activity of pain-killing biochemicals, such as endorphins and immune system cells at specific sites in the body. In addition, studies have shown that acupuncture may alter brain chemistry by changing the release of neurotransmitters and neurohormones and affecting the parts of the central nervous system related to sensation and involuntary body functions, such as immune reactions and processes whereby a person's blood pressure, blood flow, and body temperature are regulated.

Ayurvedic Medicine

Ayurveda, which literally means "the science of life," is a natural healing system developed in India. Ayurvedic texts claim that the sages who developed India's original systems of meditation and yoga developed the foundations of this medical system. It is a comprehensive system of medicine that places equal emphasis on the body, mind, and spirit, and strives to restore the innate harmony of the individual. Some of the primary Ayurvedic treatments include diet, exercise, meditation, herbs, massage, exposure to sunlight, and controlled breathing. In India, Ayurvedic treatments have been developed for various diseases (e.g., diabetes, cardiovascular conditions, and neurological disorders). However, a survey of the Indian medical literature indicates that the quality of the published clinical trials generally falls short of contemporary methodological standards with regard to criteria for randomization, sample size, and adequate controls.

Homeopathy

Homeopathy is a complete system of medical theory and practice. Its founder, German physician Samuel Christian Hahnemann (1755–1843), hypothesized that one can select therapies on the basis of how closely symptoms produced by a remedy match the symptoms of the patient's disease. He called this the "principle of similars." Hahnemann proceeded to give repeated doses of many common remedies to healthy volunteers and carefully record the symptoms they produced. This procedure is called a "proving" or, in modern homeopathy, a "human pathogenic trial." As a result of this experience, Hahnemann developed his treatments for sick patients by matching the symptoms produced by a drug to symptoms in sick patients. Hahnemann emphasized from the beginning carefully examining all aspects of a person's health status, including emotional and mental states, and tiny idiosyncratic characteristics.

> The term "homeopathy" is derived from the Greek words homeo (similar) and pathos (suffering or disease). The practice of homeopathy is based on the belief that disease symptoms can be cured by small doses of substances which produce similar symptoms in healthy people.
>
> *(Source: "CPG Sec. 400.400 Conditions Under Which Homeopathic Drugs May Be Marketed," National Cancer Institute (NCI).)*

Naturopathy

Naturopathy is a system of healing, originating from Europe, that views disease as a manifestation of alterations in the processes by which the body naturally heals itself. It emphasizes health restoration as well as disease treatment. The term "naturopathy" literally translates as "nature disease." Today naturopathy, or naturopathic medicine, is practiced throughout Europe, Australia, New Zealand, Canada, and the United States. There are six principles that form the basis of naturopathic practice in North America (not all are unique to naturopathy):

1. The healing power of nature
2. Identification and treatment of the cause of disease
3. The concept of "first do no harm"
4. The doctor as teacher
5. Treatment of the whole person
6. Prevention

The core modalities supporting these principles include diet modification and nutritional supplements, herbal medicine, acupuncture and Chinese medicine, hydrotherapy, massage and joint manipulation, and lifestyle counseling. Treatment protocols combine what the practitioner deems to be the most suitable therapies for the individual patient.

Native American Medicine

Native concepts of health and illness have sustained diverse peoples since ancient times.

Many traditional healers believe that every person has responsibility for his or her proper behavior and health, and that healing is often done by the patient. Healers therefore serve as facilitators and counselors, often using stories, humor, music, tobacco, smudging, medicinal plants and herbs, and related ceremonies to bring their healing energies into the healing space.

Chapter 9

Traditional Chinese Medicine

Traditional Chinese medicine (TCM) originated in ancient China and has evolved over thousands of years. TCM practitioners use herbal medicines and various mind and body practices, such as acupuncture and tai chi, to treat or prevent health problems. In the United States, people use TCM primarily as a complementary health approach.

Is It Safe?

- Acupuncture is generally considered safe when performed by an experienced practitioner using sterile needles. Improperly performed acupuncture can cause potentially serious side effects.
- Tai chi and qi gong, two mind and body practices used in TCM, are generally safe.

Traditional Chinese medicine (TCM) may provide short-term pain relief for temporomandibular disorders (TMD), according to a study. The study also showed that TCM may help improve quality of life. The researchers concluded that their results suggest this kind of stepped-care, community-based approach using TCM is safe and could offer short-term relief of pain and improved quality of life for patients with TMD.

(Source: "Traditional Chinese Medicine Treatment May Have Benefits For Temporomandibular Facial Pain," National Center for Complementary and Integrative Health (NCCIH).)

About This Chapter: This chapter includes text excerpted from "Traditional Chinese Medicine: In Depth," National Center for Complementary and Integrative Health (NCCIH), October 2013. Reviewed January 2018.

- There have been reports of Chinese herbal products being contaminated with drugs, toxins, or heavy metals or not containing the listed ingredients. Some of the herbs used in Chinese medicine can interact with drugs, have serious side effects, or be unsafe for people with certain medical conditions.

Is It Effective?

For most conditions, there is not enough rigorous scientific evidence to know whether TCM methods work for the conditions for which they are used.

Asthma affects millions of adults and children in the United States. Its increasing prevalence, the absence of curative treatments, and concerns about side effects from long-term use of asthma drugs have prompted interest in complementary and alternative therapies such as TCM herbs. Preliminary clinical trials of formulas containing *Radix glycyrrhizae* in combination with various other TCM herbs have had positive results. All of the trials reported improvement in lung function with the herbal formulas and found them to be safe and well tolerated.

(Source: "Time To Talk About CAM: Health Care Providers And Patients Need To Ask And Tell," National Center for Complementary and Integrative Health (NCCIH).)

Keep In Mind

Tell all your healthcare providers about any complementary health approaches you use. Give them a full picture of what you do to manage your health. This will help ensure coordinated and safe care.

Background

TCM encompasses many different practices, including acupuncture, moxibustion (burning an herb above the skin to apply heat to acupuncture points), Chinese herbal medicine, tui na (Chinese therapeutic massage), dietary therapy, and tai chi and qi gong (practices that combine specific movements or postures, coordinated breathing, and mental focus). TCM is rooted in the ancient philosophy of Taoism and dates back more than 2,500 years. Traditional systems of medicine also exist in other East and South Asian countries, including Japan (where the traditional herbal medicine is called Kampo) and Korea. Some of these systems have been influenced by TCM and are similar to it in some ways, but each has developed distinctive features of its own.

Side Effects And Risks

- Herbal medicines used in TCM are sometimes marketed in the United States as dietary supplements. The U.S. Food and Drug Administration (FDA) regulations for dietary supplements are not the same as those for prescription or over-the-counter (OTC) drugs; in general, the regulations for dietary supplements are less stringent. For example, manufacturers don't have to prove to the FDA that most claims made for dietary supplements are valid; if the product were a drug, they would have to provide proof.
- Some Chinese herbal products may be safe, but others may not be. There have been reports of products being contaminated with drugs, toxins, or heavy metals or not containing the listed ingredients. Some of the herbs used in Chinese medicine can interact with drugs, can have serious side effects, or may be unsafe for people with certain medical conditions. For example, the Chinese herb ephedra (ma huang) has been linked to serious health complications, including heart attack and stroke. In 2004, the FDA banned the sale of ephedra-containing dietary supplements, but the ban does not apply to TCM remedies.
- The FDA regulates acupuncture needles as medical devices and requires that the needles be sterile, nontoxic, and labeled for single use by qualified practitioners only. Relatively few complications from the use of acupuncture have been reported. However, adverse effects—some of them serious—have resulted from the use of nonsterile needles or improper delivery of acupuncture treatments.
- Tai chi and qi gong are considered to be generally safe practices.
- Information on the safety of other TCM methods is limited. Reported complications of moxibustion include allergic reactions, burns, and infections, but how often these events occur is not known. Both moxibustion and cupping (applying a heated cup to the skin to create a slight suction) may mark the skin, usually temporarily. The origin of these marks should be explained to healthcare providers so that they will not be mistaken for signs of disease or physical abuse.

TCM practitioners use a variety of techniques in an effort to promote health and treat disease. In the United States, the most commonly used approaches include Chinese herbal medicine, acupuncture, and tai chi.

- **Chinese herbal medicine.** The Chinese *Materia Medica* (a pharmacological reference book used by TCM practitioners) describes thousands of medicinal substances—primarily plants, but also some minerals and animal products. Different parts of plants, such as the leaves, roots, stems, flowers, and seeds, are used. In TCM, herbs are often combined in formulas and given as teas, capsules, liquid extracts, granules, or powders.

- **Acupuncture.** Acupuncture is a family of procedures involving the stimulation of specific points on the body using a variety of techniques. The acupuncture technique that has been most often studied scientifically involves penetrating the skin with thin, solid, metal needles that are manipulated by the hands or by electrical stimulation.
- **Tai chi.** Tai chi is a centuries-old mind and body practice. It involves gentle, dance-like body movements with mental focus, breathing, and relaxation.

Underlying Concepts

When thinking about ancient medical systems such as TCM, it is important to separate questions about traditional theories and concepts of health and wellness from questions about whether specific interventions might be helpful in the context of modern science-based medicine and health promotion practices.

The ancient beliefs on which TCM is based include the following:

- The human body is a miniature version of the larger, surrounding universe.
- Harmony between two opposing yet complementary forces, called *yin* and *yang*, supports health, and disease results from an imbalance between these forces.
- Five elements—fire, earth, wood, metal, and water—symbolically represent all phenomena, including the stages of human life, and explain the functioning of the body and how it changes during disease.
- Qi, a vital energy that flows through the body, performs multiple functions in maintaining health.

The Status Of TCM Research

In spite of the widespread use of TCM in China and its use in the West, rigorous scientific evidence of its effectiveness is limited. TCM can be difficult for researchers to study because its treatments are often complex and are based on ideas very different from those of modern Western medicine.

Most research studies on TCM have focused on specific techniques, primarily acupuncture and Chinese herbal remedies, and there have been many systematic reviews of studies of TCM approaches for various conditions.

- An assessment of the research found that 41 of 70 systematic reviews of the scientific evidence (including 19 of 26 reviews on acupuncture for a variety of conditions and 22 of 42 reviews on Chinese herbal medicine) were unable to reach conclusions about whether the technique worked for the condition under investigation because there was not enough good-quality evidence. The other 29 systematic reviews (including 7 of 26 reviews on acupuncture and 20 of 42 reviews on Chinese herbal medicine) suggested possible benefits but could not reach definite conclusions because of the small quantity or poor quality of the studies.
- In an analysis that combined data on individual participants in 29 studies of acupuncture for pain, patients who received acupuncture for back or neck pain, osteoarthritis, or chronic headache had better pain relief than those who did not receive acupuncture. However, in the same analysis, when actual acupuncture was compared with simulated acupuncture (a sham procedure that resembles acupuncture but in which the needles do not penetrate the skin or penetrate it only slightly), the difference in pain relief between the two treatments was much smaller—so small that it may not have been meaningful to patients.
- Tai chi has not been investigated as extensively as acupuncture or Chinese herbal medicine, but recent studies, including some supported by National Center for Complementary and Integrative Health (NCCIH), suggest that practicing tai chi may help to improve balance and stability in people with Parkinson disease; reduce pain from knee osteoarthritis and fibromyalgia; and promote quality of life and mood in people with heart failure.

If You Are Thinking About Using TCM

- Do not use TCM to replace effective conventional care or as a reason to postpone seeing a healthcare provider about a medical problem.
- Look for published research studies on TCM for the health condition that interests you.
- It is better to use TCM herbal remedies under the supervision of your healthcare provider or a professional trained in herbal medicine than to try to treat yourself.
- Ask about the training and experience of the TCM practitioner you are considering.
- If you are pregnant or nursing, or are thinking of using TCM to treat a child, you should be especially sure to consult your (or the child's) healthcare provider.
- Tell all your healthcare providers about any complementary health approaches you use. Give them a full picture of what you do to manage your health. This will help ensure coordinated and safe care.

Chapter 10

Ayurvedic Medicine

Ayurvedic medicine (also called Ayurveda) is one of the world's oldest medical systems. It originated in India more than 3,000 years ago and remains one of the country's traditional healthcare systems. Its concepts about health and disease promote the use of herbal compounds, special diets, and other unique health practices. India's government and other institutes throughout the world support clinical and laboratory research on Ayurvedic medicine, within the context of the Eastern belief system. But Ayurvedic medicine isn't widely studied as part of conventional (Western) medicine.

Is Ayurvedic Medicine Safe?

Ayurvedic medicine uses a variety of products and practices. Some of these products—which may contain herbs, minerals, or metals—may be harmful, particularly if used improperly

Advice For Consumers

- Be aware that Ayurvedic products do not undergo U.S. Food and Drug Administration (FDA) review. In accordance with current law, FDA does not evaluate these products before they are marketed. This means their safety, quality, and effectiveness cannot be assured by FDA. Certain populations, including children, are particularly at risk for the toxic effects of heavy metals.
- Tell your healthcare professional about all alternative products. Some herbs, minerals, and metals can interact with each other and with conventional medications.

(Source: "Use Caution With Ayurvedic Products," U.S. Food and Drug Administration (FDA).)

About This Chapter: This chapter includes text excerpted from "Ayurvedic Medicine: In Depth," National Center for Complementary and Integrative Health (NCCIH), January 2015.

or without the direction of a trained practitioner. For example, some herbs can cause side effects or interact with conventional medicines. Also, ingesting some metals, such as lead, can be poisonous.

Is Ayurvedic Medicine Effective

Studies have examined Ayurvedic medicine, including herbal products, for specific conditions. However, there aren't enough well-controlled clinical trials and systematic research reviews—the gold standard for Western medical research—to prove that the approaches are beneficial.

Keep In Mind

Tell all your healthcare providers about any complementary and integrative health approaches you use. Give them a full picture of what you do to manage your health. This will help ensure coordinated and safe care.

What Is Ayurveda?

The term "Ayurveda" combines the Sanskrit words *ayur* (life) and *veda* (science or knowledge). Ayurvedic medicine, as practiced in India, is one of the oldest systems of medicine in the world. Many Ayurvedic practices predate written records and were handed down by word of mouth. Three ancient books known as the Great Trilogy were written in Sanskrit more than 2,000 years ago and are considered the main texts on Ayurvedic medicine—*Caraka Samhita, Sushruta Samhita*, and *Astanga Hridaya.*

Key concepts of Ayurvedic medicine include universal interconnectedness (among people, their health, and the universe), the body's constitution *(prakriti)*, and life forces *(dosha)*, which are often compared to the biologic humors of the ancient Greek system. Using these concepts, Ayurvedic physicians prescribe individualized treatments, including compounds of herbs or proprietary ingredients, and diet, exercise, and lifestyle recommendations.

The majority of India's population uses Ayurvedic medicine exclusively or combined with conventional Western medicine, and it's practiced in varying forms in Southeast Asia.

What The Science Says About The Safety And Side Effects Of Ayurvedic Medicine

Ayurvedic medicine uses a variety of products and practices. Ayurvedic products are made either of herbs only or a combination of herbs, metals, minerals, or other materials in an

Ayurvedic practice called *rasa shastra*. Some of these products may be harmful if used improperly or without the direction of a trained practitioner.

Toxicity

Ayurvedic products have the potential to be toxic. Many materials used in them haven't been studied for safety in controlled clinical trials. In the United States, Ayurvedic products are regulated as dietary supplements. As such, they aren't required to meet the same safety and effectiveness standards as conventional medicines.

A National Center for Complementary and Integrative Health (NCCIH)-funded study examined the content of 193 Ayurvedic products purchased over the Internet and manufactured in either the United States or India. The researchers found that 21 percent of the products contained levels of lead, mercury, and/or arsenic that exceeded the standards for acceptable daily intake.

Other approaches used in Ayurvedic medicine, such as massage, special diets, and cleansing techniques may have side effects as well. To help ensure coordinated and safe care, it's important to tell all your healthcare providers about any Ayurvedic products and practices or other complementary and integrative health approaches you use.

What The Science Says About The Effectiveness Of Ayurvedic Medicine Research

Most clinical trials of Ayurvedic approaches have been small, had problems with research designs, or lacked appropriate control groups, potentially affecting research results.

- Researchers have studied Ayurvedic approaches for schizophrenia and for diabetes; however, scientific evidence for its effectiveness for these diseases is inconclusive.
- A preliminary clinical trial funded in part by NCCIH, found that conventional and Ayurvedic treatments for rheumatoid arthritis had similar effectiveness. The conventional drug tested was methotrexate and the Ayurvedic treatment included 40 herbal compounds.
- Ayurvedic practitioners use turmeric for inflammatory conditions, among other disorders. Evidence from clinical trials show that turmeric may help with certain digestive disorders and arthritis, but the research is limited.
- Varieties of boswellia (*Boswellia serrata*, *Boswellia carterii*, also known as frankincense) produce a resin that has shown anti-inflammatory and immune system effects in

laboratory studies. A preliminary clinical trial found that osteoarthritis patients receiving a compound derived from *B. serrata* gum resin had greater decreases in pain compared to patients receiving a placebo.

Chapter 11

Homeopathic Medicine

Homeopathy, also known as homeopathic medicine, is an alternative medical system that was developed in Germany more than 200 years ago.

The alternative medical system of homeopathy was developed in Germany at the end of the 18th century. Supporters of homeopathy point to two unconventional theories: "like cures like"—the notion that a disease can be cured by a substance that produces similar symptoms in healthy people; and "law of minimum dose"—the notion that the lower the dose of the

What Is Homeopathy Based On?

Homeopathy is generally based on two main principles:

- that a substance that causes symptoms in a healthy person can be used in diluted form to treat symptoms and illnesses, a principle known as "like-cures-like"; and
- the more diluted the substance, the more potent it is, which is known as the "law of infinitesimals."

Historically, homeopathic products have been identified through "provings," in which substances are administered to healthy volunteers in concentrations that cause symptoms. Symptoms experienced by volunteers are recorded to indicate possible therapeutic uses for the substances. In other words, if a substance causes a particular symptom, individuals experiencing that symptom would be treated with a diluted solution made from that substance.

(Source: "Homeopathic Products," U.S. Food and Drug Administration (FDA).)

About This Chapter: This chapter includes text excerpted from "Homeopathy," National Center for Complementary and Integrative Health (NCCIH), April 2015.

medication, the greater its effectiveness. Many homeopathic remedies are so diluted that no molecules of the original substance remain.

Homeopathic remedies are derived from substances that come from plants, minerals, or animals, such as red onion, arnica (mountain herb), crushed whole bees, white arsenic, poison ivy, belladonna (deadly nightshade), and stinging nettle. Homeopathic remedies are often formulated as sugar pellets to be placed under the tongue; they may also be in other forms, such as ointments, gels, drops, creams, and tablets. Treatments are "individualized" or tailored to each person—it is not uncommon for different people with the same condition to receive different treatments.

Regulation Of Homeopathic Treatments

Homeopathic remedies are regulated as drugs under the Federal Food, Drug and Cosmetic Act (FD&C Act). However, under current Agency policy, U.S. Food and Drug Administration (FDA) does not evaluate the remedies for safety or effectiveness.

FDA allows homeopathic remedies that meet certain conditions to be marketed without agency preapproval. For example, homeopathic remedies must contain active ingredients that are listed in the Homeopathic Pharmacopeia of the United States (HPUS). The HPUS lists active ingredients that may be legally included in homeopathic products and standards for strength, quality, and purity of that ingredient. In addition, the FDA requires that the label on the product, outer container, or accompanying leaflet include at least one major indication (i.e., medical problem to be treated), a list of ingredients, the number of times the active ingredient was diluted, and directions for use. If a homeopathic remedy claims to treat a serious disease such as cancer, it must be sold by prescription. Only products for minor health problems, like a cold or headache, which go away on their own, can be sold without a prescription.

The Status Of Homeopathy Research

Most rigorous clinical trials and systematic analyses of the research on homeopathy have concluded that there is little evidence to support homeopathy as an effective treatment for any specific condition.

A comprehensive assessment of evidence by the Australian government's National Health and Medical Research Council (NHMRC) concluded that there are no health conditions for which there is reliable evidence that homeopathy is effective.

Homeopathy is a controversial topic in complementary medicine research. A number of the key concepts of homeopathy are not consistent with fundamental concepts of chemistry and physics. For example, it is not possible to explain in scientific terms how a remedy containing little or no active ingredient can have any effect. This, in turn, creates major challenges to rigorous clinical investigation of homeopathic remedies. For example, one cannot confirm that an extremely dilute remedy contains what is listed on the label, or develop objective measures that show effects of extremely dilute remedies in the human body.

Another research challenge is that homeopathic treatments are highly individualized, and there is no uniform prescribing standard for homeopathic practitioners. There are hundreds of different homeopathic remedies, which can be prescribed in a variety of different dilutions for thousands of symptoms.

Side Effects And Risks

- Certain homeopathic products (called "nosodes" or "homeopathic immunizations") have been promoted by some as substitutes for conventional immunizations, but data to support such claims is lacking. The National Center for Complementary and Integrative Health (NCCIH) supports the Centers for Disease Control and Prevention's (CDC) recommendations for immunizations/vaccinations.
- While many homeopathic remedies are highly diluted, some products sold or labeled as homeopathic may not be highly diluted; they can contain substantial amounts of active ingredients. Like any drug or dietary supplement that contains chemical ingredients, these homeopathic products may cause side effects or drug interactions. Negative health effects from homeopathic products of this type have been reported.
- A systematic review found that highly diluted homeopathic remedies, taken under the supervision of trained professionals, are generally safe and unlikely to cause severe adverse reactions. However, like any drug or dietary supplement, these products could pose risks if they are improperly manufactured (for example, if they are contaminated with microorganisms or incorrectly diluted).
- A systematic review of case reports and case series concluded that using certain homeopathic treatments (such as those containing heavy metals like mercury or iron that are not highly diluted) or replacing an effective conventional treatment with an ineffective homeopathic one can cause adverse effects, some of which may be serious.
- Liquid homeopathic remedies may contain alcohol. The FDA allows higher levels of alcohol in these remedies than it allows in conventional drugs.

- Homeopathic practitioners expect some of their patients to experience "homeopathic aggravation" (a temporary worsening of existing symptoms after taking a homeopathic prescription). Researchers have not found much evidence of this reaction in clinical studies; however, research on homeopathic aggravations is scarce. Always discuss changes in your symptoms with your healthcare provider.
- The FDA has warned consumers about different products labeled as homeopathic. For example, in 2015, it warned consumers not to rely on asthma products labeled as homeopathic that are sold over-the-counter. These products have not been evaluated by the FDA for safety and effectiveness.

If You Are Thinking About Using Homeopathy

Do not use homeopathy as a replacement for proven conventional care or to postpone seeing a healthcare provider about a medical problem.

If you are considering using a homeopathic remedy, bring the product with you when you visit your healthcare provider. The provider may be able to help you determine whether the product might pose a risk of side effects or drug interactions.

Follow the recommended conventional immunization schedules for children and adults. Do not use homeopathic products as a substitute for conventional immunizations.

Women who are pregnant or nursing, or people who are thinking of using homeopathy to treat a child, should consult their (or their child's) healthcare providers.

Tell all your healthcare providers about any complementary health practices you use. Give them a full picture of all you do to manage your health. This will ensure coordinated and safe care.

Licensing And Certification

Laws regulating the practice of homeopathy in the United States vary from state to state. Usually, individuals who are licensed to practice medicine or another healthcare profession can legally practice homeopathy. In some states, nonlicensed professionals may practice homeopathy.

Arizona, Connecticut, and Nevada are the only states with homeopathic licensing boards for doctors of medicine (holders of M.D. degrees) and doctors of osteopathic medicine (holders of D.O. degrees). Arizona and Nevada also license homeopathic assistants, who are allowed to perform medical services under the supervision of a homeopathic physician. Some states explicitly include homeopathy within the scope of practice of chiropractic, naturopathy, and physical therapy.

Chapter 12

Native American Medicine

Native American medicine refers to the healing practices used by the indigenous peoples of North America. Native American medicine originated thousands of years ago, and it encompasses the traditions and beliefs of more than 500 distinct nations that inhabited the continent before the arrival of Europeans. One of the distinguishing features of Native American medicine is its emphasis on spiritual harmony or balance as a key component of individual health.

Native American healers typically employ a holistic approach that not only addresses the patient's specific illness or injury, but also seeks to restore the patient's spirit to a state of harmonious balance with the larger world. They view humans as part of a complex, interrelated spiritual web that encompasses the individual, the community, the Creator, and the natural environment. They believe that diseases, trauma, and bad luck are indications that the relationship between these elements has been disrupted. To return a patient to good health, a healer must also restore the balance.

Although the general thrust of Native American medicine is clear, the specific techniques and practices are not well known. Since most Native American cultures never developed a written language, healing techniques were usually passed down verbally from one generation to the next. In the centuries following European contact, many Native American nations experienced dramatic population losses as a result of warfare and epidemics of unfamiliar diseases like smallpox and measles. As traditional healers died, they often took their knowledge of Native American medicine with them.

The main documentation of Native American medicine was done by people outside of the cultural tradition. Although these people could observe and describe the physical practices,

---

they could not necessarily understand and capture their underlying spiritual meaning. In fact, some Native American healers claim that their medical practices cannot be reduced to an academic body of knowledge and technique. In addition, many Native American elders decline requests to share their healing secrets with non-natives, out of concern that their sacred practices will be dishonored or exploited and their spiritual power weakened. Some of the knowledge has survived, however, and Native American medicine continues to be practiced in the 21st century.

Healers

The traditional healers in Native American tribes were known as medicine men and medicine women. They mixed herbs and administered remedies to people who were sick or injured. In addition to practicing medicine, however, the healers were also religious leaders who helped maintain the connection between the tribe and the Creator or Great Spirit. Under the Native American belief system, an illness could have any number of different causes, including demons and evil spirits. The healers often wore grotesque masks to frighten away evil spirits and performed special ceremonies to purge the patient of demonic influences.

Most healers used tools made from natural sources, such as bones, crystals, feathers, fur, roots, shells, skin, and stones. These tools were used in ceremonies to invoke the help of the Great Spirit in healing illnesses and driving away evil. Many healers carried medicines tied in a cloth bundle or thick hide. The contents of these medicine bags were known only to the healer and were considered a sacred source of power.

Each healer was believed to have a unique perspective that grew out of their own individual skills, abilities, and life experiences. A person in need of medical treatment would seek a healer who had successfully treated other patients with similar conditions. The healer typically established a relationship with each patient in order to gain an understanding of their unique circumstances and preferences. Often the treatment was designed not only to cure a disease, but also to help the patient achieve spiritual growth and find a healthier balance with the larger world.

Healing Practices And Ceremonies

Although the healing methods used by various Native Americans nations differed, herbal remedies played a major role in medical treatment for all the tribes. Healers collected plants from surrounding areas that were known to be effective in treating certain ailments. They even traded over long distances to obtain herbs that were not available locally. Various herbs could be ground into powders to be inhaled, mashed into pastes to be applied to skin, or mixed with water or food to be consumed.

Native American healers also conducted special purification rituals, such as sweat lodges and sweat baths, to help remove toxins from a sick person's body. During these rituals, the healer usually prayed, chanted, sang, or played drums to help cleanse the body and increase clarity of thought. Sage, an herb that was believed to have powerful cleansing properties, was burned in a ceremony called "sweeping the smoke" in order to purify the body and soul.

Native American medicine also involved healing rituals and ceremonies in which the entire community participated. Rather than curing an individual patient, many of these rituals were intended to help restore harmony between the tribe and the Great Spirit in order to promote general health and prosperity. The ceremonies, which sometimes took place over several days, might involve prayers, songs and stories, chants, drumming, and various sacred healing objects. Some tribes used the medicine wheel or sacred hoop, which denotes the circle of life. It incorporates the four directions as well as Mother Earth and Father Sky.

Native American Medicine Today

In the late 1800s, the U.S. government instituted bans on Native American religious practices, which white officials considered "heathen" rituals that interfered with their goal of "civilizing" the tribes. Since these practices were closely linked to Native American medicine, many traditional healing rituals were prohibited or strongly discouraged as well. After being suppressed for decades, many ancient medical practices were forgotten. Meanwhile, in the early 20th century the federal Indian Health Service began opening hospitals and clinics on reservations to bring modern medicine to Native American communities. An increasing number of Native Americans turned to these facilities for their heath care needs, especially to treat "white man's diseases" that their healers had proven unable to cure.

The passage of the American Indian Religious Freedom Act in 1978 finally lifted the federal ban on Native American religious practices and healing rituals. Since then, mainstream medical theory has shifted toward a more holistic approach that recognizes a patient's mental and spiritual well-being as an important component of their physical health. As a result, Native American medicine has experienced a surge in popularity and interest in recent years.

Traditional herbal remedies drawn from Native American traditions, for instance, hold strong appeal for people who are concerned about the toxicity, addictive properties, and side effects of pharmaceutical drugs. Some people believe that these natural remedies, which have been developed over centuries, can be as effective as prescription medications in treating certain conditions.

Many Native American communities face serious health concerns in the 21st century, including high rates of alcoholism, obesity, diabetes, and heart disease. While most Native Americans rely on conventional medicine to treat these health problems, many find that traditional healing practices provide benefits as well. In addition, the holistic approach used by Native American healers has increasingly attracted non-native adherents. By treating the patient's body, mind, and spirit together, they believe that Native American medicine can improve their chances of healing and maintaining good health.

References

1. Center for Health and Healing. "Traditional and Indigenous Healing Systems: Native American Medicine," Mt. Sinai Beth Israel, 2003.
2. Mehl-Madrona, Lewis. "Traditional (Native American) Indian Medicine Treatment of Chronic Illness," Healing Center Online, 2008.
3. Weiser, Kathy. "Native American Medicine," Legends of America, May 2015.

Chapter 13

Naturopathy

Naturopathy—also called naturopathic medicine—is a medical system that has evolved from a combination of traditional practices and healthcare approaches popular in Europe during the 19th century.

People visit naturopathic practitioners for various health related purposes, including primary care, overall well-being, and treatment of illnesses.

In the United States, naturopathy is practiced by naturopathic physicians, traditional naturopaths, and other healthcare providers who also offer naturopathic services.

What Naturopathic Practitioners Do

Naturopathic practitioners use many different treatment approaches. Examples include:

- Dietary and lifestyle changes
- Exercise therapy
- Herbs and other dietary supplements
- Homeopathy
- Manipulative therapies
- Practitioner guided detoxification
- Psychotherapy and counseling
- Stress reduction

About This Chapter: This chapter includes text excerpted from "Naturopathy," National Center for Complementary and Integrative Health (NCCIH), September 24, 2017.

Some practitioners use other methods as well or, if appropriate, may refer patients to conventional healthcare providers.

Detoxification

A variety of "detoxification" ("detox") diets and regimens—also called "cleanses" or "flushes"—have been suggested as a means of removing toxins from your body or losing weight. Detoxification may be promoted in many settings and may also be used in naturopathic treatment.

(Source: "Detoxes And Cleanses," National Center for Complementary and Integrative Health (NCCIH).)

Education And Licensure Of Practitioners

Education and licensing differ for the three types of naturopathic practitioners:

- **Naturopathic physicians** generally complete a 4-year, graduate level program at one of the North American naturopathic medical schools accredited by the Council on Naturopathic Medical Education (CNME), an organization recognized for accreditation purposes by the U.S. Department of Education (ED). Some U.S. states and territories have licensing requirements for naturopathic physicians; others don't. In those jurisdictions that have licensing requirements, naturopathic physicians must graduate from a 4-year naturopathic medical college and pass an examination to receive a license. They must also fulfill annual continuing education requirements.
- **Traditional naturopaths,** also known simply as "naturopaths," may receive training in a variety of ways. Training programs vary in length and content and are not accredited by organizations recognized for accreditation purposes by the ED. Traditional naturopaths are often not eligible for licensing.
- **Other healthcare providers** (such as physicians, osteopathic physicians, chiropractors, dentists, and nurses) sometimes offer naturopathic treatments, functional medicine, and other holistic therapies, having pursued additional training in these areas. Training programs vary.

Remember that regulations, licenses, or certificates do not guarantee safe, effective treatment from any healthcare provider—conventional or complementary.

Tell all your healthcare providers about any complementary or integrative health approaches you use. Give them a full picture of what you do to manage your health. This will help ensure coordinated and safe care.

Chapter 14

Osteopathy

What Is Osteopathy?

Osteopathy was developed as a drug-free, noninvasive form of healthcare that recognizes the important link between body structure and function. This system aims to improve an individual's health by strengthening the musculoskeletal framework, so osteopathic procedures focus on a person's joints, muscles, and spine. Techniques such as moving, stretching, gentle pressure, and resistance are known as osteopathic manipulative medicine (OMM). The principle behind this treatment is that an individual's well-being depends on the muscles, ligaments, bones, and connective tissues working together harmoniously.

Osteopathy was established as a method of treatment by an American physician, Andrew Taylor Still, in 1874. Still rejected many common medical practices of the day, such as bloodletting and narcotic sedation, which often did more harm than good, believing instead that the human body could be helped to heal itself through noninvasive and nonmedicinal means. He studied many alternative theories and experimented with a variety of treatments, finally coming to the conclusion that correct musculoskeletal alignment is the key to good health. He also taught proper health maintenance and is credited with being one of the first doctors to promote preventative care.

At present, osteopathy is one of the fastest growing professions in the United States and is widely regarded as a complementary therapy used alongside more conventional methods to help treat disease and improve health. In the United States, osteopathic physicians (DOs) are trained and function as medical doctors (MDs). They use the same medical techniques as other physicians but tend to take a more holistic approach to healthcare. In other parts of the

---

world, this is not necessarily the case, so practitioners of osteopathy may function differently and receive different kinds of training.

Before undergoing any treatment by an osteopathic physician, the patient should ensure that the doctor is certified by the American Osteopathic Association (AOA) and is a licensed practitioner. A display of documentation in his or her practice is necessary. The patient's regular doctor, if any, should be kept in the loop when osteopathic treatment is undertaken.

How Is It Performed?

Osteopathic treatment is very patient-centric, and an initial consultation generally takes place before any treatment begins. The doctor asks about the patient's general health, current medications, symptoms, and any other medical care received. After the consultation, the osteopathic physician will examine the patient physically, possibly using his or her hands to find areas of weakness, tenderness, or strain within the body. The patient may be asked to do certain stretches and movements to allow the physician to observe the patient's posture and range of motion. Depending on the patient's health requirements, the physician may prescribe a plan for treatment that will encompass several sessions. The patient may also be asked to make some dietary and lifestyle changes to get the best results from osteopathy.

Doctors trained in osteopathy can identify whether a patient needs further testing, such as blood tests or a magnetic resonance imaging (MRI) scan, to help diagnose the health issue better.

Cost of the treatment varies depending on the clinic, insurance plan, and the state. Note that an osteopathic physician differs from a chiropractor. Although both pay special attention to bone and muscle structures, a chiropractor is not a medical doctor and focuses only on a specific problem area, while an osteopathic physician deals with the body as a whole.

Osteopathic Techniques

Traditional osteopathic treatment concentrates on restoring the stability of the joints to return the body to health. Osteopathic physicians frequently use their hands for treatment, which includes a mixture of gentle and forceful techniques, some of which include:

- **Articulation.** The joints are moved through a natural range of motion.
- **Stretching.** Stiff joints are stretched.
- **Massaging.** Manipulation is done to relax the muscles.

- **High-Velocity Thrusts.** These are quick, sharp movements to the spine that may produce a sound like the cracking of knuckles.

These techniques are intended to help to increase blood flow, improve movement, and ease pain. Osteopathic treatments are generally pain-free; however, afterwards some patients experience a degree of soreness or stiffness, particularly if the treatment is done for a painful or inflamed injury. Patients are advised to inform the osteopathic physician if any pain is experienced during the treatment. Some exercises may be recommended by the physician for faster recovery.

Benefits Of Osteopathy

Osteopathy can be especially beneficial for patients who have conditions that affect their muscles, joints, and bones. Some of them include:

- sports injuries
- pelvis, hip, and leg problems
- neck pain
- shoulder pain
- arthritis
- lower back pain
- postural problem

Osteopathic treatments can strengthen the musculoskeletal framework and other systems. Today's lifestyle, especially sitting and lack of exercise, can lead to a variety of musculoskeletal problems, including lower back pain. In such cases, the physician may use gentle manipulation to stretch and massage the muscles. In addition to osteopathic treatments, the doctor might also discuss a number of preventative methods that can help. Osteopathic treatment has also been shown to reduce insomnia since pain and discomfort in muscles and joints can lead to a sleepless night.

Risks Of Osteopathy

Osteopathy can involve a few risks. Stiffness after the treatment is common in many patients for a couple of days, and some may also experience headaches. A few less common side effects include rib fractures, severe pain, tingling, and numbness. Very rare, more serious adverse effects, such as stroke, nerve damage, muscle weakness, bladder problems, and prolapsed disk, require immediate medical attention. Patients should be made aware of these risks before the treatment begins.

References

1. "About Osteopathy," Canadian College of Osteopathy, January 15, 2016.
2. Nordqvist, Christian. "Everything You Need to Know about Osteopathy," Medical News Today, July 5, 2017.
3. "Osteopathy," NHS Choices, November 11, 2011.

Part Three
Manipulative Practices And Movement Therapies

Chapter 15

Chiropractic Medicine

Chiropractic is a healthcare profession that focuses on the relationship between the body's structure—mainly the spine—and its functioning. Although practitioners may use a variety of treatment approaches, they primarily perform adjustments (manipulations) to the spine or other parts of the body with the goal of correcting alignment problems, alleviating pain, improving function, and supporting the body's natural ability to heal itself.

The term "chiropractic" combines the Greek words cheir (hand) and praxis (practice) to describe a treatment done by hand. Hands-on therapy—especially adjustment of the spine—is central to chiropractic care. Chiropractic is based on the notion that the relationship between the body's structure (primarily that of the spine) and its function (as coordinated by the nervous system) affects health.

Spinal adjustment/manipulation is a core treatment in chiropractic care, but it is not synonymous with chiropractic. Chiropractors commonly use other treatments in addition to spinal manipulation, and other healthcare providers (e.g., physical therapists or some osteopathic physicians) may use spinal manipulation.

Use In The United States

In the United States, chiropractic is often considered a complementary health approach. According to the National Health Interview Survey (NHIS), which included a comprehensive survey of the use of complementary health approaches by Americans, about 8 percent of adults

About This Chapter: This chapter includes text excerpted from "Chiropractic: In Depth," National Center for Complementary and Integrative Health (NCCIH), February 2012. Reviewed January 2018.

(more than 18 million) and nearly 3 percent of children (more than 2 million) had received chiropractic or osteopathic manipulation in the past 12 months. Additionally, an analysis of NHIS cost data found that adults in the United States spent approximately $11.9 billion out-of-pocket on visits to complementary health practitioners—$3.9 billion of which was spent on visits to practitioners for chiropractic or osteopathic manipulation.

Many people who seek chiropractic care have low-back pain. People also commonly seek chiropractic care for other kinds of musculoskeletal pain (e.g., neck, shoulder), headaches, and extremity (e.g., hand or foot) problems.

An analysis of the use of complementary health approaches for back pain, based on data from the NHIS, found that chiropractic was by far the most commonly used therapy. Among survey respondents who had used any of these therapies for their back pain, 74 percent (approximately 4 million Americans) had used chiropractic. Among those who had used chiropractic for back pain, 66 percent perceived "great benefit" from their treatments.

In one study funded by National Center for Complementary and Integrative Health (NCCIH) that examined long-term effects in more than 600 people with low-back pain, results suggested that chiropractic care involving spinal manipulation was at least as effective as conventional medical care for up to 18 months.

(Source: "Spinal Manipulation For Low-Back Pain," National Center for Complementary and Integrative Health (NCCIH).)

Treatment

During the initial visit, chiropractors typically take a health history and perform a physical examination, with a special emphasis on the spine. Other examinations or tests such as X-rays may also be performed. If chiropractic treatment is considered appropriate, a treatment plan will be developed.

During follow-up visits, practitioners may perform one or more of the many different types of adjustments and other manual therapies used in chiropractic care. Given mainly to the spine, a chiropractic adjustment involves using the hands or a device to apply a controlled, rapid force to a joint. The goal is to increase the range and quality of motion in the area being treated and to aid in restoring health. Joint mobilization is another type of manual therapy that may be used.

Chiropractors may combine the use of spinal adjustments and other manual therapies with several other treatments and approaches such as:

- Heat and ice
- Electrical stimulation
- Relaxation techniques
- Rehabilitative and general exercise
- Dietary supplements
- Counseling about diet, weight loss, and other lifestyle factors

What The Science Says

Researchers have studied spinal manipulation for a number of conditions ranging from back, neck, and shoulder pain to asthma, carpal tunnel syndrome, fibromyalgia, and headaches. Much of the research has focused on low-back pain, and has shown that spinal manipulation appears to benefit some people with this condition.

A review of scientific evidence on manual therapies for a range of conditions concluded that spinal manipulation/mobilization may be helpful for several conditions in addition to back pain, including migraine and cervicogenic (neck-related) headaches, neck pain, upper- and lower-extremity joint conditions, and whiplash-associated disorders. The review also identified a number of conditions for which spinal manipulation/mobilization appears not to be helpful (including asthma, hypertension, and menstrual pain) or the evidence is inconclusive (e.g., fibromyalgia, mid-back pain, premenstrual syndrome, sciatica, and temporomandibular joint disorders).

Safety

- Side effects from spinal manipulation can include temporary headaches, tiredness, or discomfort in the parts of the body that were treated.
- There have been rare reports of serious complications such as stroke, cauda equina syndrome (a condition involving pinched nerves in the lower part of the spinal canal), and worsening of herniated discs, although cause and effect are unclear.
- Safety remains an important focus of ongoing research:
    - A study of treatment outcomes for 19,722 chiropractic patients in the United Kingdom concluded that minor side effects (such as temporary soreness) after cervical

spine manipulation were relatively common, but that the risk of a serious adverse event was "low to very low" immediately or up to 7 days after treatment.

- A study that drew on 9 years of hospitalization records for the population of Ontario, Canada analyzed 818 cases of vertebrobasilar artery (VBA) stroke (involving the arteries that supply blood to the back of the brain). The study found an association between visits to a healthcare practitioner and subsequent VBA stroke, but there was no evidence that visiting a chiropractor put people at greater risk than visiting a primary care physician. The researchers attributed the association between healthcare visits and VBA stroke to the likelihood that people with VBA dissection (torn arteries) seek care for related headache and neck pain before their stroke.

Practitioners: Education And Licensure

Chiropractic colleges accredited by the Council on Chiropractic Education (CCE) offer Doctor of Chiropractic (D.C.) degree programs. (CCE is the agency certified by the U.S. Department of Education (ED) to accredit chiropractic colleges in the United States.) Admission to a chiropractic college requires a minimum of 90 semester hour credits of undergraduate study, mostly in the sciences.

Chiropractic training is a 4-year academic program that includes both classroom work and direct experience caring for patients. Coursework typically includes instruction in the biomedical sciences, as well as in public health and research methods. Some chiropractors pursue a 2- to 3-year residency for training in specialized fields.

Chiropractic is regulated individually by each state and the District of Columbia. All states require completion of a Doctor of Chiropractic degree program from a CCE-accredited college. Examinations administered by the National Board of Chiropractic Examiners (NBCE) are required for licensing and include a mock patient encounter. Most states require chiropractors to earn annual continuing education credits to maintain their licenses. Chiropractors' scope of practice varies by state in areas such as the dispensing or selling of dietary supplements and the use of other complementary health approaches such as acupuncture or homeopathy.

If You Are Thinking About Seeking Chiropractic Care

- Ask about the chiropractor's education and licensure.
- Mention any medical conditions you have, and ask whether the chiropractor has specialized training or experience in the condition for which you are seeking care.

- Ask about typical out-of-pocket costs and insurance coverage. (Chiropractic is covered by many health maintenance organizations and private health plans, Medicare, and state workers' compensation systems.)
- Tell the chiropractor about any medications (prescription or over-the-counter (OTC)) and dietary supplemcnts you take. If the chiropractor suggests a dietary supplement, ask about potential interactions with your medications or other supplements.
- Tell all of your healthcare providers about any complementary health approaches you use. Give them a full picture of what you do to manage your health. This will help ensure coordinated and safe care.

Chapter 16

Kinesiotherapy

History Of Kinesiotherapy

Kinesiotherapy (KT) is the application of scientifically based exercise principles adapted to enhance the strength, endurance, coordination, range of motion, and mobility of individuals with functional limitations or those requiring extended physical conditioning. Kinesiotherapy (formerly corrective therapy) is an allied health profession whose origins can be traced back to 1943.

The roots of this profession began during World War II when corrective physical reconditioning units were established to accelerate the return of urgently needed troops to active duty following injury. Corrective therapists, as a result, became a part of the U.S. Armed Forces' rehabilitation effort employing exercise and mobility programming. As the demand for these physical reconditioning specialists grew, early leaders in rehabilitation recognized the need to organize and accredit these new specialists accordingly through a structured educational curriculum.

Since that time, the discipline has expanded into both the public and private sectors. At present, the U.S. Department of Veterans Affairs (VA) is the single largest employer of kinesiotherapists providing services to Service members through a holistic approach to overall patient care emphasizing the psychological as well as physical benefits of therapeutic exercise

About This Chapter: Text under the heading "History Of Kinesiotherapy" is excerpted from "Kinesiotherapist At Richmond VA Medical Center," U.S. Department of Veterans Affairs (VA), September 10, 2013. Reviewed January 2018; Text under the heading "What Kinesiotherapist Do" is excerpted from "Kinesiotherapist," U.S. Bureau of Labor Statistics (BLS), U.S. Department of Labor (DOL), December 2014. Reviewed January 2018; Text beginning with the heading "Treatment Settings" is excerpted from "Kinesiotherapy Fact Sheet," U.S. Department of Veterans Affairs (VA), January 2015.

and education within the acute and post-acute rehabilitation process. Kinesiotherapists apply advanced skills, certifications, and specialty training in their practice across the continuum of care for members with a wide spectrum of neurologic, orthopedic, mental health, surgical, and medical conditions, including special populations such as stroke, spinal cord injury, traumatic brain injury (TBI), amputation, homeless, and geriatric patients. Advanced skills include, but not limited to, driver rehabilitation, cardiopulmonary rehabilitation, geriatric rehabilitation, psychiatric rehabilitation, polytrauma rehabilitation, prosthetic, orthotic and amputation rehabilitation as well as functional capacity evaluations, therapeutic aquatics, wheelchair seating, and spinal cord injury rehabilitation.

What Kinesiotherapist Do

Job duties for kinesiotherapists vary, depending on where they work—and sometimes within the facility itself. Responsibilities usually include assessing and treating patients, among other tasks.

Kinesiotherapists work under a physician's direction, often with other specialists, such as a nurse, a dietitian, and a social worker.

Assessment

To determine what exercises and training may be beneficial, a kinesiotherapist first evaluates patients to assess their physical abilities and activity levels. This assessment allows the kinesiotherapist to decide how much help, if any, patients need each day for routine tasks, such as walking, eating, and getting into and out of bed.

Home-care providers also do an environmental assessment of the patient's residence to ensure safety. This includes evaluating a home's potential safety risks—such as stairs, unsafe furniture, and nonworking smoke detectors—and recommending corrective action.

Treatment

Kinesiotherapists base a patient's treatment plan on what they learned during assessment. Emphasizing the physical and psychological benefits of exercise, they focus on reconditioning and physical education. Treatment is tailored to each patient's needs and situation.

For example, Laura Hines a kinesiotherapist had a patient with mobility problems who was limited to crawling in his own home. The patient could stand for only brief periods, so Laura created a plan that would help him rebuild strength gradually. "I started him on a treadmill for a few minutes at a time, because he needed to rest in between," she says. Eventually, through reconditioning exercises with Laura's guidance, the patient became fully mobile not just inside his house but out and about as well.

Other Duties

In addition to tasks related to assessment and treatment, kinesiotherapists have some administrative duties. These include documenting patient visits; ordering equipment, such as adaptive-eating utensils or wheelchairs; and participating in outreach activities.

Some kinesiotherapists' other responsibilities are related to the work but specific to their patient population.

Treatment Settings

Kinesiotherapy provides a full scope of services. Treatment settings include inpatient settings (including medical centers and community living centers), outpatient clinics, and telerehabilitation.

Kinesiotherapy Training

Kinesiotherapists are highly trained healthcare professionals. Entry-level education requirements include a bachelor's degree in kinesiotherapy or exercise science with an emphasis in kinesiotherapy. This education must include or be supplemented by clinical practice in a VA approved training program or its equivalent.

Kinesiotherapy promotes an environment for clinical education. There are on average, about 60 KT students participating in clinical internship across the VHA each year.

Clinical Training Partnerships

The Council on Professional Standards for Kinesiotherapy (COPS-KT) signed a Memorandum of Understanding (MoU) on January 31, 2012 to begin clinical training for masters prepared exercise science majors who have completed the core educational requirements in kinesiotherapy.

Advanced Training

Many Kinesiotherapists have advanced skills, certification and training in specialty areas. Advanced skills include driver rehabilitation, cardiopulmonary rehabilitation, geriatrics, orthopedics, polytrauma, and amputation. Kinesiotherapy advanced training also includes functional capacity evaluations, therapeutic aquatics, wheelchair seating, and spinal cord injury (SCI).

Evidence-Based Medicine

Kinesiotherapists provide state-of-the-art and evidence-based care to Service members. VA's provision of evidence-based medical and rehabilitation care is supported through a system-wide collaboration with Joint Commission, and Commission on Accreditation of Rehabilitation Facilities (CARF) to achieve and maintain national accreditation for VA Acute Care and Rehabilitation Programs.

Chapter 17

Lymphatic Drainage Therapy

Lymphatic drainage therapy is a manual massage technique intended to reduce fluid buildup and swelling that may occur due to problems with the lymph nodes. Lymph is a clear, watery fluid that flows through a network of tissues, organs, and vessels known as the lymphatic system. The main components of the lymphatic system include the bone marrow, spleen, and thymus, as well as lymph nodes located in the neck, armpits, chest, and groin.

The lymph nodes play a vital role in the functioning of the immune system. They filter out harmful substances that are carried in the lymph fluid, such as bacteria and viruses, and attack and destroy them with white blood cells called lymphocytes. If a person has an infection, injury, or a disease like cancer, the lymph nodes may become tender and swollen as they aid in the immune response.

When the lymph nodes are compromised by disease or surgically removed, the lymphatic system may lose its ability to drain fluid from a nearby region of the body, resulting in a condition called lymphedema. Problems involving the lymph nodes in the armpit, for instance, may result in painful fluid buildup and swelling in the arm. Lymphatic drainage therapy was developed to treat lymphedema and related conditions.

Causes And Symptoms Of Lymphedema

Lymphedema can be related to several different factors. Primary lymphedema, which is rare, can arise at birth as a result of a malformed or dysfunctional lymphatic system. The more common condition, secondary lymphedema, can result from anything that obstructs or causes damage to the lymphatic system, including infection, injury, cancer, surgery, or radiation therapy.

Among the most common causes of secondary lymphedema are cancer and cancer treatments. When surgeons operate to remove a malignancy, they often remove lymph nodes in the area of the tumor to determine whether cancer cells are present in the lymphatic system. If the cancer has spread to the lymph nodes, the patient faces a higher risk that the disease will come back following surgery. The degree to which the cancer has affected the lymph nodes determines its stage of advancement and the type of treatment that the patient requires. Cancer in the lymph nodes, surgical removal of the lymph nodes, and radiation therapy designed to kill cancer cells can all cause lymphedema.

Regardless of the cause, the symptoms of lymphedema include swelling of the hands, arms, feet, legs, or any other part of the body; loss of mobility in the affected joints and limbs; redness, itching, and tightening of the skin; and general feelings of heaviness and discomfort.

Massage Therapy For Lymph Drainage

Chronic lymphedema has no cure, but there are a number of methods that can be used to help manage its severity and symptoms. One option is lymphatic drainage or manual massage therapy. Developed in Europe in the 1930s, it is intended to improve the natural flow of lymph and the drainage of fluids from body parts affected by lymphedema.

The manual massage technique involves gentle rubbing, tapping, and stroking of the skin using a specific speed, pressure, and pattern. The goal is to stimulate the movement of lymph out of congested areas, bypassing the damaged lymph vessels, and channel it into healthy vessels so that it can return to systemic circulation.

Manual massage treatments should begin with a certified therapist, although patients can learn to perform the technique on themselves. Generally, it does not involve risks when done correctly. However, the technique should not be used on open wounds, broken skin, or tissues that have been exposed to radiation therapy. It is also not suitable if the patient has a deep vein thrombosis (blood clot).

Proponents claim that manual massage therapy can lead to improvements in many different medical conditions, including poor circulation, injuries, burns, nervous system disorders, arthritis, pregnancy-related swelling, varicose veins, stress, and insomnia. A few studies have indicated that women with lymphedema related to breast cancer treatment may experience a reduction in swelling following manual massage therapy. But the efficacy of the treatment must be demonstrated in larger, controlled studies for it to gain acceptance in the mainstream medical community.

References

1. American Cancer Society. "Lymph Nodes and Cancer," 2015.
2. Dr. Vodder School International. "Manual Lymphatic Drainage," 2015.
3. National Cancer Institute. "Lymphedema for Health Professionals: Manual Lymphedema Therapy," 2015.

Chapter 18

Massage Therapy

Many people associate massage with vacations or spas and consider them something of a luxury. But research is beginning to suggest this ancient form of hands-on healing may be more than an indulgence—may help improve your health.

What The Massage Therapists Do

Massage therapists use their fingers, hands, forearms and elbows to manipulate the muscles and other soft tissues of the body. Variations in focus and technique lead to different types of massage, including Swedish, deep tissue, and sports massage.

In Swedish massage, the focus is general and the therapist may use long strokes, kneading, deep circular movements, vibration, and tapping. With a deep tissue massage, the focus is more targeted, as therapists work on specific areas of concern or pain. These areas may have muscle "knots" or places of tissue restriction.

Why Do People Go For Massage Therapy?

Some common reasons for getting a massage are to relieve pain, heal sports injuries, reduce stress, relax, ease anxiety or depression, and aid general wellness.

About This Chapter: Text in this chapter begins with excerpts from "Massage Therapy—What You Knead To Know," *NIH News in Health,* National Institutes of Health (NIH), July 2012. Reviewed January 2018; Text beginning with the heading "What The Science Says About The Effectiveness Of Massage" is excerpted from "Massage Therapy For Health Purposes," National Center for Complementary and Integrative Health (NCCIH), June 2016.

What The Science Says About The Effectiveness Of Massage

A lot of the scientific research on massage therapy is preliminary or conflicting, but much of the evidence points toward beneficial effects on pain and other symptoms associated with a number of different conditions. Much of the evidence suggests that these effects are short term and that people need to keep getting massages for the benefits to continue.

Researchers have studied the effects of massage for many conditions. Some that they have studied more extensively are the following:

Pain

- A research review and National Center for Complementary and Integrative Health (NCCIH)-funded clinical trial concluded that massage may be useful for chronic low-back pain.
- Massage may help with chronic neck pain, a NCCIH-funded clinical trial reported.
- Massage may help with pain due to osteoarthritis of the knee, according to a NCCIH-funded study.
- Studies suggest that for women in labor, massage provided some pain relief and increased their satisfaction with other forms of pain relief, but the evidence isn't strong, a review concluded.

Cancer

Numerous research reviews and clinical studies have suggested that at least for the short term, massage therapy for cancer patients may reduce pain, promote relaxation, and boost mood. However, the National Cancer Institute (NCI) urges massage therapists to take specific precautions with cancer patients and avoid massaging:

- Open wounds, bruises, or areas with skin breakdown
- Directly over the tumor site
- Areas with a blood clot in a vein
- Sensitive areas following radiation therapy

Mental Health

- A meta-analysis of 17 clinical trials concluded that massage therapy may help to reduce depression.
- Brief, twice-weekly yoga and massage sessions for 12 weeks were associated with a decrease in depression, anxiety, and back and leg pain in pregnant women with depression, a NCCIH-funded clinical trial showed. Also, the women's babies weighed more than babies born to women who didn't receive the therapy.
- However, a research review concluded that there's not enough evidence to determine if massage helps pregnant mothers with depression.
- A review concluded that massage may help older people relax.
- For generalized anxiety disorder (GAD), massage therapy was no better at reducing symptoms than providing a relaxing environment and deep breathing lessons, according to a small, NCCIH-supported clinical trial.

Fibromyalgia

A review concluded that massage therapy may help temporarily reduce pain, fatigue, and other symptoms associated with fibromyalgia, but the evidence is not definitive. Researchers noted that it's important that the massage therapist not cause pain.

Headaches

Clinical trials on the effects of massage for headaches are preliminary and only somewhat promising.

Human Immunodeficiency Virus (HIV) / Acquired Immunodeficiency Syndrome (AIDS)

Massage therapy may help improve the quality of life for people with HIV or AIDS, a review of four small clinical trials concluded.

Infant Care

Massaging preterm infants using moderate pressure may improve weight gain, a review suggested. Researchers don't have enough evidence to know if massage benefits healthy infants who are developing normally, a review determined.

Other Conditions

Researchers have studied massage for the following but it's still unclear if it helps:

- Behavior of children with autism or autism spectrum disorders
- Immune function in women with breast cancer
- Anxiety and pain in patients following heart surgery
- Quality of life and glucose levels in people with diabetes
- Lung function in children with asthma

What The Science Says About The Safety And Side Effects Of Massage Therapy

Massage therapy appears to have few risks when performed by a trained practitioner. However, massage therapists should take some precautions in people with certain health conditions.

Whom You Should Consult Before Considering Massage Therapy

If you're considering massage therapy for a specific medical condition, talk with your healthcare provider. Never use massage to replace your regular medical care or as a reason to postpone seeing a healthcare professional.

Every therapist and every massage is unique. If you decide to try massage therapy, work with different therapists until you find one that meets your needs. One of the best ways to get a great massage is to communicate with your therapist. Most will check in with you during your session for feedback, but—if not—speak up!

(Source: "Massage Therapy—What You Knead To Know," NIH News in Health, *National Institutes of Health (NIH).)*

- In some cases, pregnant women should avoid massage therapy. Talk with your healthcare provider before getting a massage if you're pregnant.
- People with some conditions such as bleeding disorders or low blood platelet counts should avoid having forceful and deep tissue massage. People who take anticoagulants

(also known as blood thinners) also should avoid them. Massage should not be done in any potentially weak area of the skin, such as wounds.

- Deep or intense pressure should not be used over an area where the patient has a tumor or cancer, unless approved by the patient's healthcare provider."

Chapter 19

Reflexology (Zone Therapy)

Reflexology is based on the idea that applying pressure to specific points on the feet, hands, or ears will produce beneficial effects on the corresponding body organs and a person's general health. It is utilized worldwide as a complementary and alternative treatment method for a variety of conditions, such as anxiety, asthma, cancer, diabetes, headaches, premenstrual syndrome, and stress.

Reflexology is also known as zone therapy. According to proponents of the method, the body is divided into ten longitudinal zones, with five located on each side of the body. Each zone within the body is represented by a certain point on the hands or feet. Practitioners claim to be able to detect abnormalities in the organs of each zone by feeling the corresponding areas on the hands or feet. Once the problem has been identified, the reflexologist puts pressure on the reflex points in order to stimulate a flow of energy, blood, nutrients, and nerve impulses to the zone.

Reflexology has experienced a rapid increase in popularity in Europe and Asia. In several countries, in fact, local governing bodies and private companies have begun employing reflexologists to treat their staff members. The practice has been credited with helping to increase job satisfaction and reduce absenteeism in some of these organizations.

Origin And Development Of Reflexology

Reflexology has been practiced since ancient times. It is depicted in a pictograph on the Egyptian tomb of Ankhamor that dates to 2330 BCE, for instance, as well as in symbols engraved on the feet of Buddha statues in India and China. The earliest discussion of reflexology in print appears in the *Yellow Emperor's Classic of Internal Medicine,* a Chinese text written around 1,000 BCE. Marco Polo is credited with introducing reflexology methods in Europe in the 1300s by translating Chinese massage instructions into Italian.

The so-called Father of Zone Therapy in the United States was Dr. William H. Fitzgerald. In 1913, he introduced the idea that putting pressure on certain points on the feet and hands could exert an anaesthetic effect on other parts of the body. He used the zone therapy technique to relieve pain from injuries or minor medical procedures. Fitzgerald's work was expanded by Dr. Shelby Riley, who also suggested pressure points on the outer ear. Another important contribution was made by Eunice D. Ingham, a physiotherapist who mapped the body's reflex zones in the 1940s.

Reflexology Points And Areas

Although the practice of reflexology varies in different parts of the world, most practitioners agree on the major reflex points. Reflexologists use maps to represent the correspondence between these points on the feet, hands, and ears and different bodily systems. Each foot represents a vertical half of the body, for instance, with points on the left foot corresponding to organs on the left side of the body and points on the right foot corresponding to organs on the right side of the body. For instance, the liver, which is located on the right side of the abdomen, is represented by an area on the right foot.

Research On Reflexology

Medical research into the effectiveness of reflexology has yielded mixed results. Most patients find reflexology therapy relaxing, and many report that it provides such health benefits as relieving pain, reducing anxiety, improving mood, and enhancing sleep. Studies funded by the U.S. National Institutes of Health have supported the anecdotal evidence that reflexology may help alleviate pain and reduce the psychological stress associated with injury and illness. As a result, reflexology treatments are increasingly being used as part of the palliative care of people with cancer.

On the other hand, the mainstream medical community generally rejects the idea that reflexology can effectively diagnose and treat potentially serious medical conditions, such as asthma, diabetes, or cancer. A 2009 systematic review of controlled studies concluded that reflexology had failed to demonstrate effectiveness in treating any medical condition. Critics argue that there is no scientific evidence to support claims that reflexology practitioners can identify problems or improve the function of bodily systems by putting pressure on reflex points. They point out that medical research has never established any nerve connection or flow of energy between reflex points and other parts of the body.

Although reflexology is not considered harmful and may aid some patients with the psychological aspects of healing, doctors warn that it should only be used in addition to, rather than in place of, appropriate medical treatment.

References

1. Barrett, Stephen. "Reflexology: A Close Look," Quackwatch, 2015.
2. Bauer, Brent A. "What Is Reflexology? Can It Relieve Stress?" Mayo Clinic, 2015.
3. Teagarden, Karen. "Reflexology," *Taking Charge of Your Health and Well-Being,* University of Minnesota Center for Spirituality and Healing, 2013.

Chapter 20

Spinal Manipulation

Low-back pain (often referred to as "lower back pain") is a common condition that usually improves with self-care (practices that people can do by themselves, such as remaining active, applying heat, and taking pain-relieving medications). However, it is occasionally difficult to treat. Some healthcare professionals are trained to use a technique called spinal manipulation to relieve low-back pain and improve physical function (the ability to walk and move).

About Low-Back Pain

Back pain is one of the most common health complaints, affecting 8 out of 10 people at some point during their lives. The lower back is the area most often affected. For many people, back pain goes away on its own after a few days or weeks. But for others, the pain becomes chronic and lasts for months or years. Low-back pain can be debilitating, and it is a challenging condition to diagnose, treat, and study. The total annual costs of low-back pain in the United States—including lost wages and reduced productivity—are more than $100 billion.

About Spinal Manipulation

Spinal manipulation—sometimes called "spinal manipulative therapy"—is practiced by healthcare professionals such as chiropractors, osteopathic physicians, naturopathic physicians, physical therapists, and some medical doctors. Practitioners perform spinal manipulation by using their hands or a device to apply a controlled force to a joint of the spine. The amount of force applied depends on the form of manipulation used. The goal of the treatment is to relieve pain and improve physical functioning.

About This Chapter: This chapter includes text excerpted from "Spinal Manipulation For Low-Back Pain," National Center for Complementary and Integrative Health (NCCIH), April 2013. Reviewed January 2018.

A clinical trial has added to knowledge about what goes on in the body and brain when people with chronic low-back pain receive spinal manipulation (also known as spinal manipulative therapy). The researchers found that spinal manipulation, compared with placebo and no treatment, significantly reduced pain sensitivity. They also reported there was support for a potential biological target to address central sensitization of pain, a phenomenon of heightened pain sensitivity that is linked with acute pain's transition to chronic pain, and the persistence of chronic pain.

(Source: "Spinal Manipulation's Effects May Go Beyond Those Of Placebo Or Expectation, Study Finds," National Center for Complementary and Integrative Health (NCCIH).)

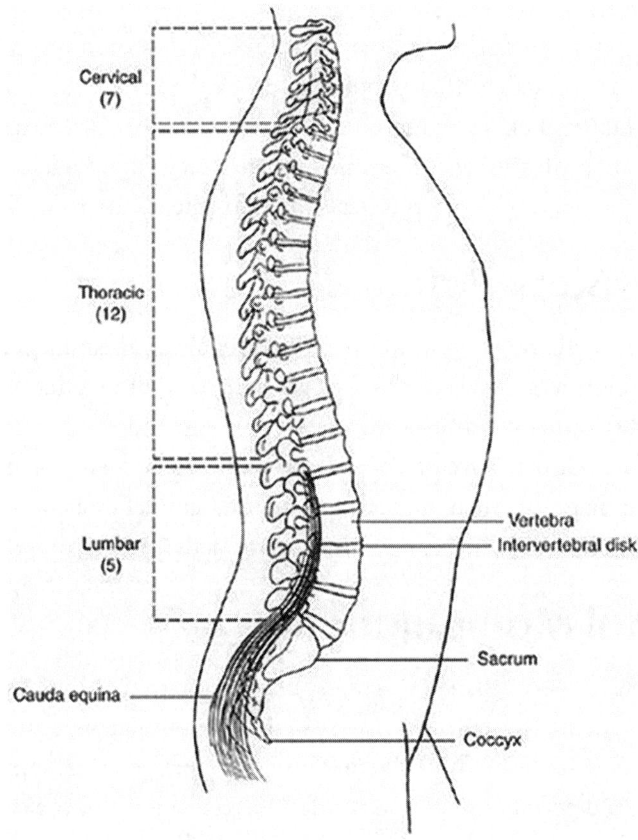

Figure 20.1. Side View Of Spine

(Source: "Back Pain," National Institute of Arthritis and Musculoskeletal and Skin Diseases (NIAMS).)

Side Effects And Risks

Reviews have concluded that spinal manipulation for low-back pain is relatively safe when performed by a trained and licensed practitioner. The most common side effects are generally minor and include feeling tired or temporary soreness.

Reports indicate that CES, a significant narrowing of the lower part of the spinal canal in which nerves become pinched and may cause pain, weakness, loss of feeling in one or both legs, and bowel or bladder problems, may be an extremely rare complication of spinal manipulation. However, it is unclear if there is actually an association between spinal manipulation and CES, since CES usually occurs without spinal manipulation. In people whose pain is caused by a herniated disc, manipulation of the low back appears to have a very low chance of worsening the herniation.

What The Science Says About Spinal Manipulation For Low-Back Pain

Overall, studies have shown that spinal manipulation is one of several options—including exercise, massage, and physical therapy—that can provide mild-to-moderate relief from low-back pain. Spinal manipulation also appears to work as well as conventional treatments such as applying heat, using a firm mattress, and taking pain-relieving medications.

The American College of Physicians (ACP) and the American Pain Society (APS) included spinal manipulation as one of several treatment options for practitioners to consider when low-back pain does not improve with self-care. An Agency for Healthcare Research and Quality (AHRQ) report noted that complementary health therapies, including spinal manipulation, offer additional options to conventional treatments, which often have limited benefit in managing back and neck pain. The AHRQ analysis also found that spinal manipulation was more effective than placebo and as effective as medication in reducing low-back pain intensity. However, the researchers noted inconsistent results when they compared spinal manipulation with massage or physical therapy to reduce low-back pain intensity or disability.

Researchers continue to study spinal manipulation for low-back pain.

- A review of 26 clinical trials looked at the effectiveness of different treatments, including spinal manipulation, for chronic low-back pain. The researchers concluded that spinal manipulation is as effective as other interventions for reducing pain and improving function.

- A review that looked at various manual therapies, such as spinal manipulation and massage, for a range of conditions found strong evidence that spinal manipulation is effective for chronic low-back pain and moderate evidence of its effectiveness for acute low-back pain.
- An analysis looked at the evidence from 76 trials that studied the effects of several conventional and complementary health practices for low-back pain. The researchers found that the pain-relieving effects of many treatments, including spinal manipulation, were small and were similar in people with acute or chronic pain.
- A review that focused on spinal manipulation for chronic low-back pain found strong evidence that spinal manipulation works as well as a combination of medical care and exercise instruction, moderate evidence that spinal manipulation combined with strengthening exercises works as well as prescription nonsteroidal anti-inflammatory drugs combined with exercises, and limited-to-moderate evidence that spinal manipulation works better than physical therapy and home exercise.

Researchers are investigating whether the effects of spinal manipulation depend on the length and frequency of treatment. In one study funded by National Center for Complementary and Integrative Health (NCCIH) that examined long-term effects in more than 600 people with low-back pain, results suggested that chiropractic care involving spinal manipulation was at least as effective as conventional medical care for up to 18 months. However, less than 20 percent of participants in this study were pain-free at 18 months, regardless of the type of treatment used.

Researchers are also exploring how spinal manipulation affects the body. In an NCCIH-funded study of a small group of people with low-back pain, spinal manipulation affected pain perception in specific ways that other therapies (stationary bicycle and low-back extension exercises) did not.

Chapter 21

Rolfing Structural Integration

What Is Rolfing Structural Integration (SI)?

Rolfing® is a system of movement education and body manipulation that reorganizes connective tissues, known as fascia. The connective tissues support, stabilize, and surround all the muscles, nerves, bones, and organs in the body. The system aims to align the entire body with the Earth's gravity by manipulating the particular fascia that affect posture and structure in a positive manner. The Rolfing method does not see the body as a collection of separate parts, but rather a network of connected tissues and works on them to realign, release, and balance the whole body. The main goal of Rolfing structural integration (SI) is to restore flexibility, revitalize energy, and help one regain balance and vitality.

Structural Integration (SI): Procedure

Structural Integration (SI) is an alternative method of manual therapy and somatosensory training that purports to improve biomechanical functioning of the body as a whole rather than to focus on the treatment of specific symptoms. SI therapists employ both manipulation and somatosensory education. SI is delivered in a series of ten treatments, referred to as "the Ten Series," each of approximately one hour in duration. The Ten Series protocol includes manipulation of all major joints and anatomical segments. Each of the ten sessions aims to achieve a different set of biomechanical changes, which are regarded as contributing to the progressive approximation of specific ideals of posture and movement.

(Source: "Structural Integration For Chronic Low Back Pain," ClinicalTrials.gov, National Institutes of Health (NIH).)

Origin Of Rolfing SI

Rolfing SI was named after its founder, Dr. Ida P. Rolf. In 1920, she received her doctorate in biochemistry from Columbia University and furthered her study of the human body through her work in organic chemistry at the Rockefeller Institute. Her interest and research were mainly oriented towards methods that emphasized the effect of structure on function, such as osteopathy, yoga, and chiropractic. Rolf combined her research with other scientific knowledge about the body's structural order to develop Rolfing SI and began practicing the technique on clients.

During her lifetime, Rolf taught her methods to many students at the Esalen Institute in Big Sur, California, and since her death in 1979, these students and other practitioners have continued to use the methods and expand on them. At present, this method is practiced in about 27 countries, and there are more than 1,200 certified Rolfers worldwide. Although there have been few objective scientific studies validating the effectiveness of Rolfing, through the years many thousands of individuals claim to have benefited from structural integration.

How Does Rolfing SI Work?

The system aims to align and balance body structures until the entire body functions and coordinates smoothly. Its primary focus is on the fascial system, which is like an internal wire-network for the entire body. If something goes wrong, such as one set of wires being out of place or becoming rigid, the result can be sore muscles, joint pain, or a shift in posture. The Rolfing method tries to ease tension and bring back balance and alignment to the entire body. Rolf's insights led her to believe that when body structures are balanced in gravity, they function more effectively and remain at ease.

If there are internal misalignments, the Rolfing system uses mild, direct pressure to release tension in the fascia and allow for rejuvenation of health through the re-establishment of balance. The deep, slow strokes of Rolfing stimulate intra-fascial mechanoreceptors that enable the nervous system to be triggered and reduce strain on the muscles.

Rolfing SI seeks to restore alignment to body systems that are out of place. For example, when positioned correctly the legs are aligned to the hips, shoulders to the rib cage, and joints and related tissue are integrated into one another with the body positioned over the feet. The Rolfing method allows the healthy level of muscle contraction to be established and alleviates pain.

How Does Rolfing Differ From Massage?

Although Rolfing involves hands-on manipulation by a practitioner, it differs from deep tissue massage. While massage is purely aimed at relaxing the muscles, Rolfing seeks to improve body alignment and functionality. It concentrates on and affects body posture and structure for longer periods. The method may also speed up recovery from injury, rigid muscle tension, movement around joints, and any secondary pain.

Rolfing is typically administered via "The Ten," a series of ten sessions divided into three groups or units. The first group strives to loosen surface layers of connective tissue in the shoulders, arms, ribcage, spine, hips, and feet. The next unit concentrates on the core area between the pelvis and the head. And the final group of sessions focuses on progress made in previous steps and integrating a sense of permanent order and balance in the body.

Benefits Of Rolfing SI

Some of the major benefits attributing to Rolfing are listed below.

- People have experienced a reduction in pain, improved flexibility and posture, as well as a deep sense of body awareness with the Rolfing method.
- Rolfing can permanently alter a person's posture, stability, and structure.
- The Rolfing method restores balance to the body by releasing unnecessary tension.
- An estimated one million people have undergone Rolfing treatment, including dancers, athletes, and businesspeople.
- Proponents say that Rolfing results in the more efficient use of muscles, helps the body conserve energy, and creates refined patterns of movement.
- Rolfing is said to help neurological function and reduce the spinal misalignment of individuals with lordosis, or curvature of the spine.

Who Should Use Rolfing SI?

Dr. Rolf had a global vision that imagined a more structurally efficient human species through the application of Rolfing. Therefore, she believed all children and adults should receive Rolfing SI since all bodies have some degree of disorder and imbalance. People with a history of injury or trauma from accidents and people with minor injuries that interfere with their daily activities are also said to benefit from the method. People without injuries also can use Rolfing because it is intended to help enhance overall body functionality and condition. It is also said to have helped some people attain enhanced spiritual and emotional well-being.

References

1. "How Does Rolfing Structural Integration Work?" Rolf Institute of Structural Integration, August 10, 2012.
2. Lynn, Judy. "Rolfing and MS: Bliss or Pain?" Multiple Sclerosis News Today, January 17, 2018.
3. "What Is Rolfing?" Action Potential, October 14, 2010.
4. "What Is Rolfing Structural Integration?" Rolf Institute of Structural Integration, September 20, 2017.

Chapter 22

Feldenkrais Method

The Feldenkrais method is a therapy system that uses movement to help people learn new and effective ways of living a holistic life. The method was developed by Moshe Feldenkrais, a physicist and engineer, who synthesized insights from biomechanics, psychology, motor development, and martial arts to develop an effective and practical application that can help people reconnect with their health through movement. Feldenkrais was born into a Hasidic family and community. A serious injury that impaired his walking prompted him to explore the connection between body movement and healing. This not only restored his ability to walk, but also led him to many breakthrough discoveries in human movement. Before his death in 1984, Feldenkrais trained about 300 practitioners to continue his work, and now around 6,000 Feldenkrais practitioners are at work around the world. The method continues to influence other disciplines, such as education, psychology, child development, sports, gerontology, and occupational therapy, and has also helped develop the new field of somatic education.

Feldenkrais method was influenced by Moshe Feldenkrais involvement in jiujister, a martial art. Feldenkrais incorporated the views of neurosurgeon Karl H. Pribram and cyberneticist Heinz Von Foerster. Esther Thelen, human development researcher also influenced Feldenkrais Method. Moshe Feldenkrais said that humans move according to their perceived self-image, so his method employs different strategies to improve posture, coordination, flexibility, and athletic ability. It also intended to help relieve chronic pain, restricted movement, back pain, and other common ailments. Neurological and psychological problems are also resolved using this type of therapy. The Feldenkrais method employs new ways of moving by expanding one's perception and awareness to enable a person to be more aware of his or her habits and body tension and move accordingly.

The Feldenkrais method teaches that personal history, cultural background, upbringing, injuries, and illness make people adopt a set of behaviors, both physical and psychological. Sometimes these behaviors become so dysfunctional or outmoded that they get embedded deep into the nervous system and create unnecessary physical and psychological limitations. It analyses the person's cultural and biological aspects of movement, posture, learning, and habits to see how they limit his or her potential. The method also engages organic learning and movement to enable freedom from habitual patterns and allows new methods of movement, thinking, and feeling to emerge.

The Feldenkrais method is taught in two formats:

- Functional Integration (FI)
- Awareness Through Movement (ATM)

Functional Integration (FI)

Functional integration (FI), also known as Feldenkrais private sessions, is a one-to-one approach between the teacher and individual student. The teacher helps the student in movement lessons through gentle and noninvasive touch as the primary means of communication. The FI lessons are quite flexible, allowing the student to take it at his or her own pace and as their needs demand. The lessons are done by the student sitting, standing, or lying on a specially designed table. The teacher uses touch to reflect how the student organizes current body movements and patterns. The instructor then analyses and teaches more effective movement patterns for the student. The teacher creates a comfortable environment for the student so that learning becomes easier, then focuses on the student's abilities and needs, with more forceful procedures being employed as necessary.

FI lessons relate to how much a student desires to learn, their intent, and their need for the lesson. The lessons are customized according to the student's unique requirements, and they learn how to integrate the learned movements into their daily lives. FI is a gentle and subtle method widely recognized to heal minor aches and pains, musculoskeletal problems, neurological problems, tension, and child developmental issues.

Awareness Through Movement (ATM)

Similar to tai chi or gentle yoga, Awareness Through Movement (ATM) reengages the nervous system. People usually pick up certain habits and behaviors when they are infants and later abandon them. Through ATM, the old habits are replaced by new skills and awareness through engaging a person's entire body. ATM is generally taught in group classes in which students walk, stand, sit, or lie on the floor as the instructor takes them through a series of carefully planned movements intended to retrain neuromuscular patterns.

References

1. "About Feldenkrais Method," The Feldenkrais Institute, April 30, 2009.
2. "About the Feldenkrais Method," Feldenkrais.com, June 17, 2017.
3. "Feldenkrais Method," Goodtherapy.org, July 19, 2016.
4. Fry, Rich. "The Feldenkrais Method," Flowingbody.com, n.d.

Chapter 23

The Alexander Technique

The Alexander Technique is an educational method that helps individuals learn to relieve harmful tension in their bodies by correcting faulty movement and posture habits. This method has been used for more than 100 years and is said to be a unique and effective technique of mind-body reeducation. The process identifies patterns and movements that are inefficient and result in the accumulation of tension. It is not a set of passive treatments but a method for changing how one thinks and responds.

> People who learn the Alexander Technique report feeling more vibrant, relaxed, and stable.

The technique was created by Frederick Matthias Alexander, an Australian teacher and actor. It began as a method for singers and actors to improve their vocal training. But Alexander discovered that the basis for all vocal education was dependent on developing a highly efficient respiratory system, which led him to focus his process on the breathing mechanism. Some students who had come to Alexander for vocal training recognized that their respiratory difficulties were getting better over time. The improvements were periodically noted by medical doctors and eventually led to the refinement of the Alexander Technique.

Basic Concepts Of The Alexander Technique

In his writings, Alexander laid out the terminology for his method's basic concepts:

- **Primary control.** Alexander called the relationship between the head, neck, and back primary control. He believed that this relationship was critical in determining overall body function and movement.

- **Recognizing a habit.** Over the years people develop certain habits, some good and others bad. A teacher who is trained in the Alexander Technique helps students recognize these habits in order to begin changing them for the better.
- **Direction.** Humans have an innate ability to send messages from the brain to the muscles through the nervous system. The Alexander Technique shows how this ability can be used to promote better muscular function.
- **Inhibition.** Individuals react automatically and habitually to stimuli. The Alexander Technique aims to train students to use the gap between stimulus and response to choose a productive course of action. Alexander called this inhibition because students are taught to circumvent, or inhibit, their habitual responses.
- **Faulty sensory appreciation.** Certain habits can affect the accuracy of kinesthetic feedback that may prevent an individual from making positive change. The first step in initiating correction is being taught to recognize these faulty habits.

Learning The Alexander Technique

Proponents of the Alexander Technique say that it is a practical and unique way of stopping or changing detrimental habits. Students learn to refrain from habitual patterns that are not useful and develop movements that are natural and spontaneous. The teacher guides the students through movement, coordination patterns, and posture and helps them visualize their body movements. The learning procedure helps students gain a natural perspective about their own sense of coordination. The teacher uses verbal and gentle hands-on guidance to enable the students to experience natural and easy movements without the interference of their current habits. When the process is repeated and expanded, the students' internal coordination becomes more accurate. This helps them respond to stimuli in a coordinated and nonstressful manner.

Advantages Of The Alexander Technique

Teachers, students, and other advocates of the Alexander Technique have identified a number of benefits of the method:

- **Improved posture.** By recognizing habits that hinder normal and spontaneous movements and unlearning habits caused by tension, the Alexander Technique enables individuals to develop and maintain good posture.

- **Skill enhancement.** Many professionals, like athletes and performing artists, use the Alexander Technique to improve their performance in their respective fields.
- **Pain relief.** The technique can help identify and unlearn habitual patterns that lead to musculoskeletal pain caused by excess tension. People tend to tense up during episodes of pain which further aggravates the condition. The technique is said to help relieve neck, back, and joint pain for long periods.
- **Ability to deal with stress.** The technique teaches individuals to deal with any anxiety-producing stimulus by using unique movements designed to reduce tension and empower an individual to handle pressure more effectively.

Efficacy Of The Alexander Technique

The Alexander technique is a method that teaches people how to stop using high levels of muscular and mental tension during their everyday activities. Twenty four weekly lessons in Alexander technique were shown to improve Parkinson disease (PD) patients' own assessment of their disability at the end of lessons, and when reassessed 6 months later. Compared with PD patients who received no treatment, those receiving Alexander technique lessons were less depressed by the end of the lessons. Alexander technique is currently recommended for PD patients by the National Institute for Health and Clinical Evidence (United Kingdom).

(Source: "Alternative Therapies For Parkinson's Disease," U.S. Department of Veterans Affairs (VA).)

References

1. "Alexander Technique," Health & Wellness, University of New Hampshire, n.d.
2. "Alexander Technique: The Insider's Guide," Alexander Technique Center of Washington, February 1, 2002.
3. "Frequently Asked Questions: Alexander Technique Basics," American Society for the Alexander Technique, September 28, 2010.
4. "What Is the Alexander Technique: What Are the Benefits of Lessons or Classes?" The Complete Guide to the Alexander Technique, March 16, 2012.

Part Four
Mind-Body Medicine

Chapter 24

About Mind-Body Medicine

Mind And Body Practice

A health practice that combines mental focus, controlled breathing, and body movements to help relax the body and mind. It may be used to help control pain, stress, anxiety, and depression, and for overall health. Examples of mind-body practices include meditation, hypnosis, guided imagery, yoga, and tai chi. A mind-body practice is a type of complementary and alternative medicine (CAM). It is also called mind-body modality.

Today

- A National Health Interview Survey (NHIS) found that 19.2 percent of American adults and 4.3 percent of children aged 17 and younger had used at least one CAM mind-body therapy in the year prior to the survey.
- Pain was the most common reason for CAM use in this survey.
- Many studies document that psychological stress is linked to a variety of health problems, such as increased heart disease, compromised immune system functioning, and premature cellular and cognitive aging. Some evidence suggests that mind-body therapies could reduce psychological stress.

About This Chapter: Text under the heading "Mind And Body Practice" is excerpted from "NCI Dictionary Of Cancer Terms," National Cancer Institute (NCI), June 15, 2012. Reviewed January 2018; Text beginning with the heading "Today" is excerpted from "Mind-Body Medicine Practices In Complementary And Alternative Medicine," National Institutes of Health (NIH), March 29, 2013. Reviewed January 2018; Text under the heading "Seven Things To Know About Mind And Body Practices For Children And Teens" is excerpted from "7 Things To Know About Mind And Body Practices For Children And Teens," National Center for Complementary and Integrative Health (NCCIH), March 23, 2017.

- Recent results from National Institutes of Health (NIH)-funded studies on CAM mind-body therapies include:
- Pain sufferers often seek relief though CAM therapies, including mind-body modalities. A review of the evidence on various mind-body therapies to help treat certain neurological diseases involving pain found some evidence for positive effects from some therapies—including biofeedback for migraine headache, yoga for fatigue from multiple sclerosis, and relaxation therapy as a part of comprehensive programs to help control epileptic seizures.
- In a study of 60 breast cancer survivors, women who used hypnosis reduced the number and severity of hot flashes and also reported improvements in mood and sleep.
- A small preliminary trial suggests that Zen meditation may be a strategy to help prevent and/or reduce the cognitive decline of normal aging.
- A study of 63 people with rheumatoid arthritis found that Mindfulness-Based Stress Reduction (MBSR) helped to improve quality of life and reduce psychological distress.
- A study of 298 college students found that Transcendental Meditation (TM) helped students reduce stress and improve coping strategies.
- In a study of 50 women, regular practice of yoga benefited mood and physiological response to stress.
- People with fibromyalgia may benefit from practicing tai chi according to a study in 66 people. Study participants who practiced tai chi had a significantly greater decrease in total score on the Fibromyalgia Impact Questionnaire (FIQ). In addition, the tai chi group demonstrated greater improvement in sleep quality, mood, and quality of life.
- Tai chi may also be a safe alternative to conventional exercise for maintaining bone mineral density in postmenopausal women, thus helping to prevent or slow osteoporosis, increase musculoskeletal strength, and improve balance.

Tomorrow

- A research collaborative is examining how patient expectations and other factors in patient-provider interactions may produce biological effects that play a role in health outcomes. Results from this research will inform how healthcare providers relate to their patients, and will also help to explain the biological mechanisms underlying mind-body medicine.

- Obesity and metabolic syndrome are increasingly common conditions that increase risk for diabetes and cardiovascular disease. An experimental program that combines mindfulness meditation, "mindful eating," and diet/exercise may help to control these conditions. Researchers are testing whether the program improves hormonal responses to stress and aids weight control.
- A study of loving-kindness/compassion meditation and mindfulness meditation is looking at effects on the brain/body—especially regulation of emotions. Can meditation train the mind to change the brain? Findings may have applications for conditions linked with emotions and stress, such as recurrent depression.

Seven Things To Know About Mind And Body Practices For Children And Teens

Nearly 12 percent of children and teens (about one in nine) in the United States are using some form of complementary health product or practice, such as chiropractic or spinal manipulation, yoga, meditation, or massage therapy. Mind and body practices include a variety of procedures and techniques done or taught by a trained practitioner or teacher to help improve health and well-being. Older children and teens can do some mind and body activities on their own (or with help from a parent or guardian), such as relaxation techniques and deep breathing. Mind and body practices are generally safe if used appropriately, but the number of studies looking at their safety specifically for children is limited.

Here are 7 things to know about common mind and body practices for children and teens.

1. Biofeedback, guided imagery, mindfulness, and yoga are some of the mind and body practices that have the best evidence of being effective for children and are low-risk.
2. Acupuncture appears to be safe for most children, but side effects can occur if it's done by poorly trained practitioners.
3. Massage therapy appears to have few risks when done by a trained practitioner. However, massage therapists need to take extra precautions with people who have certain health conditions, such as bleeding disorders.
4. Relaxation techniques are generally safe for healthy people, including children. However, there have been rare reports that some relaxation techniques might cause or worsen symptoms in people with epilepsy or certain psychiatric conditions, or with a history of abuse or trauma.

5. Spinal manipulation is usually safe for healthy people but is also associated with rare but serious complications.
6. Follow the Centers for Disease Control and Prevention's (CDC) vaccination recommendations to safeguard your child against vaccine-preventable diseases. Vaccinating children helps protect our community's and our children's health.
7. It's important that you talk with your child's healthcare provider about any complementary health approach that you're using or considering for your child, and encourage your teenagers to do the same.

Chapter 25

Biofeedback

What Is Biofeedback?

Biofeedback is a type of therapy that helps people control certain body functions that otherwise take place involuntarily, such as blood pressure, heart rate, skin temperature, and muscle tension. The biofeedback technique works on the principle that by harnessing the power of one's mind, a person can be aware of the processes taking place inside their body, and this can give them more control over their health. With biofeedback, electrodes or sensors are attached to the skin. These help receive information about the body, measure processes, and display the results on a monitor. Using this information, a biofeedback therapist can help a person learn how the heart rate or blood pressure can be controlled. The individual then uses the monitor to see his or her progress and eventually will be able to achieve success without it. The therapy is said to prevent or treat conditions such as high blood pressure, chronic pain, migraine headaches, and urinary incontinence.

Biofeedback Methods

Depending on the individual's need, a biofeedback therapist recommends the appropriate course of action. Some biofeedback therapies include:

- **Brain wave.** This method uses scalp sensors attached to an electroencephalograph (EEG) to monitor brain waves.
- **Breathing.** Breathing patterns and respiration rate are observed by placing bands around the abdomen and chest during respiration.

- **Muscle.** Electromyography (EMG) is used to measure muscle tension. This involves placing sensors over skeletal muscles to monitor electrical activity.
- **Heart rate.** An electrocardiograph (ECG) measures the heart rate and its variability. This method of feedback uses sensors placed on the chest, wrist, or lower torso.
- **Temperature.** Blood flow to the skin is measured using sensors attached to the fingers or feet.
- **Sweat glands**. Sweat gland activity and skin perspiration are measured by an electrodermograph (EDG) by attaching sensors to the fingers, palm, or wrist.

How Does Biofeedback Work?

Biofeedback is known to promote relaxation and help relieve stress. Researchers are not sure how the method works; however, people who have undergone treatment report benefiting greatly from biofeedback therapy. When the body is under stress, certain internal processes, like blood pressure and heart rate, tend to become overactive. Biofeedback promotes relaxation, and many scientists believe that this is the key to stress reduction and other health benefits. A biofeedback therapist can help an individual learn to reduce stress through mental exercises and physical relaxation techniques.

A Biofeedback Session

A typical biofeedback session involves attaching electrodes to an individual's skin. The electrodes send signals to a monitor that displays the current heart rate, breathing rate, skin temperature, blood pressure, muscle activity, and perspiration. If the individual is under stress, muscles tighten, heart rate becomes faster, blood pressure rises, sweating increases, and breathing quickens. When the monitor displays variation from normal rates, the biofeedback therapist trains the individual to manage these functions through various mental and physical relaxation techniques. This eventually helps the individual bring involuntary internal body functions under his or her control outside of the therapy session.

The following are some of the types of relaxation techniques used in biofeedback therapy:

- **Progressive muscle relaxation.** Tightening and relaxing different muscle groups.
- **Mindfulness meditation.** Negative emotions are purged by refocusing thought processes.
- **Guided imagery.** Focusing on a specific calming image makes one feel more relaxed.
- **Deep breathing.** A breathing exercise intended to promote a sense of well-being.

Benefits Of Biofeedback

Proponents of biofeedback cite many of its benefits that can be used to manage both physical and mental issues. Biofeedback therapy is found to be most effective for conditions influenced by stress, such as eating and learning disorders, bedwetting, and muscle spasms. Other problems that can be helped by biofeedback include asthma, incontinence, irritable bowel syndrome (IBS), constipation, high blood pressure, chronic pain, anxiety, depression, diabetes, headaches, and the effects of chemotherapy. Researchers have found that biofeedback has also helped improve intelligence and behavior in children, reportedly including attention deficit hyperactivity disorder (ADHD) and autism. Some people prefer biofeedback to other types of therapy since it is noninvasive and reduces the need for medication.

EEG Biofeedback And Posttraumatic Stress Disorder (PTSD)

EEG biofeedback is an emerging alternative approach to treating posttraumatic stress disorder (PTSD), for which there is still insufficient evidence to assume unequivocal clinical utility. EEG biofeedback has also been explored as a treatment for non-PTSD related anxiety disorders, with results showing significant changes in reported anxiety correlated with increased or decreased alpha-frequency (~8–12 Hz) power. Similarly, alpha-frequency EEG biofeedback has been shown to reduce anxiety and to reduce heart rate reactivity to a stressor after 8 sessions of EEG biofeedback training.

(Source: "EEG Biofeedback Therapy As An Adjunct Treatment For PTSD," ClinicalTrials.gov, National Institutes of Health (NIH).)

Biofeedback method is more useful and effective in children. For instance, EEG neurofeedback (especially when combined with cognitive therapy) has been found to improve behavior and intelligence scores in children with attention deficit hyperactivity disorder (ADHD) and autism. Abdominal pain can be relieved by biofeedback combined with a fibre-rich diet. Migraine and chronic tension headaches among children and teens can be relieved or controlled by thermal biofeedback.

Risks Of Biofeedback

Biofeedback is generally considered safe, and research has not revealed any side effects. A consultation with a primary healthcare provider is a good idea before beginning therapy since biofeedback may not be for everyone. For example, some people with existing serious mental health issues might not find this form of treatment to be beneficial.

References

1. "Biofeedback," Mayo Clinic, January 3, 2018.
2. Kiefer, David, MD. "Overview of Biofeedback," WebMD, August 1, 2016.
3. Ehrlich, D. Steven, NMD. "Biofeedback," University of Maryland Medical Center, November 6, 2015.
4. "Biofeedback," Healthline, January 11, 2016.
5. Nordqvist, Joseph. "Biofeedback," Medical News Today, January 10, 2017.

Chapter 26

Relaxation Techniques

What Are Relaxation Techniques?

Relaxation techniques include a number of practices such as progressive relaxation, guided imagery, biofeedback, self-hypnosis, and deep breathing exercises. The goal is similar in all: to produce the body's natural relaxation response, characterized by slower breathing, lower blood pressure, and a feeling of increased well-being.

Meditation and practices that include meditation with movement, such as yoga, and tai chi, can also promote relaxation.

Stress management programs commonly include relaxation techniques. Relaxation techniques have also been studied to see whether they might be of value in managing various health problems.

To Reduce Stress

- Get enough sleep.
- Exercise regularly. Just 30 minutes a day of walking can boost mood and reduce stress.
- Build a social support network.
- Set priorities. Decide what must get done and what can wait. Say no to new tasks if they are putting you into overload.

About This Chapter: This chapter includes text excerpted from "Relaxation Techniques For Health," National Center for Complementary and Integrative Health (NCCIH), May 2016.

- Think positive. Note what you've accomplished at the end of the day, not what you've failed to do.
- Try relaxation methods. Mindfulness, meditation, yoga, or tai chi may help.
- Seek help. Talk to a mental health professional if you feel unable to cope, have suicidal thoughts, or use drugs or alcohol to cope.

(Source: "Feeling Stressed? Stress Relief Might Help Your Health," NIH News in Health, *National Institutes of Health (NIH).)*

The Importance Of Practice

Relaxation techniques are skills, and like other skills, they need practice. People who use relaxation techniques frequently are more likely to benefit from them. Regular, frequent practice is particularly important if you're using relaxation techniques to help manage a chronic health problem. Continuing use of relaxation techniques is more effective than short-term use.

What Does Relaxation Techniques Include?

Relaxation techniques includes the following:

Autogenic Training

In autogenic training, you learn to concentrate on the physical sensations of warmth, heaviness, and relaxation in different parts of your body.

Biofeedback Assisted Relaxation

Biofeedback techniques measure body functions and give you information about them so that you can learn to control them. Biofeedback assisted relaxation uses electronic devices to teach you to produce changes in your body that are associated with relaxation, such as reduced muscle tension.

Deep Breathing Or Breathing Exercises

This technique involves focusing on taking slow, deep, even breaths.

Guided Imagery

For this technique, people are taught to focus on pleasant images to replace negative or stressful feelings. Guided imagery may be self-directed or led by a practitioner or a recording.

Progressive Relaxation

This technique, also called Jacobson relaxation or progressive muscle relaxation (PMR), involves tightening and relaxing various muscle groups. Progressive relaxation is often combined with guided imagery and breathing exercises.

Self-Hypnosis

In self-hypnosis programs, people are taught to produce the relaxation response when prompted by a phrase or nonverbal cue (called a "suggestion").

What The Science Says About The Effectiveness Of Relaxation Techniques

Researchers have evaluated relaxation techniques to see whether they could play a role in managing a variety of health conditions, including the following:

Anxiety

Studies have shown relaxation techniques may reduce anxiety in people with ongoing health problems such as heart disease, or inflammatory bowel disease, and in those who are having medical procedures such as breast biopsies or dental treatment. Relaxation techniques have also been shown to be useful for older adults with anxiety.

On the other hand, relaxation techniques may not be the best way to help people with generalized anxiety disorder (GAD). GAD is a mental health condition, lasting for months or longer, in which a person is often worried or anxious about many things and finds it hard to control the anxiety. Studies indicate that long-term results are better in people with GAD who receive a type of psychotherapy called cognitive behavioral therapy (CBT) than in those who are taught relaxation techniques.

Asthma

There hasn't been enough research to show whether relaxation techniques can relieve asthma symptoms in either adults or children.

Childbirth

Relaxation techniques such as guided imagery, progressive muscle relaxation, and breathing techniques may be useful in managing labor pain. Studies have shown that women who were taught self-hypnosis have a decreased need for pain medicine during labor. Biofeedback hasn't been shown to relieve labor pain.

Depression

An evaluation of 15 studies concluded that relaxation techniques are better than no treatment in reducing symptoms of depression but are not as beneficial as psychological therapies such as CBT.

Epilepsy

There's no reliable evidence that relaxation techniques are useful in managing epilepsy.

Fibromyalgia

- Studies of guided imagery for fibromyalgia have had inconsistent results.
- A 2013 evaluation of the research concluded that electromyographic (EMG) biofeedback, in which people are taught to control and reduce muscle tension, helped to reduce fibromyalgia pain, at least for short periods of time. However, EMG biofeedback didn't affect sleep problems, depression, fatigue, or health related quality of life in people with fibromyalgia, and its long-term effects haven't been established.

Headache

- Biofeedback. Biofeedback has been studied for both tension headaches and migraines.
  - An evaluation of high quality studies concluded that there's conflicting evidence about whether biofeedback can relieve tension headaches.
  - Studies have shown decreases in the frequency of migraines in people who were using biofeedback. However, it's unclear whether biofeedback is better than a placebo.
- Other Relaxation Techniques. Relaxation techniques other than biofeedback have been studied for tension headaches. An evaluation of high-quality studies found conflicting evidence on whether relaxation techniques are better than no treatment or a placebo. Some studies suggest that other relaxation techniques are less effective than biofeedback.

Heart Disease

In people with heart disease, studies have shown relaxation techniques can reduce stress and anxiety and may also have beneficial effects on physical measures such as heart rate.

High Blood Pressure

Stress can lead to a short-term increase in blood pressure, and the relaxation response has been shown to reduce blood pressure on a short-term basis, allowing people to reduce their need for blood pressure medication. However, it's uncertain whether relaxation techniques can have long-term effects on high blood pressure.

Insomnia

There's evidence that relaxation techniques can be helpful in managing chronic insomnia. Relaxation techniques can be combined with other strategies for getting a good night's sleep, such as maintaining a consistent sleep schedule; avoiding caffeine, alcohol, heavy meals, and strenuous exercise too close to bedtime; and sleeping in a quiet, cool, dark room.

Irritable Bowel Syndrome (IBS)

An evaluation of research results by the American College of Gastroenterology (ACG) concluded that relaxation techniques have not been shown to help IBS. However, other psychological therapies, including CBT and hypnotherapy, are associated with overall symptom improvement in people with IBS.

Menstrual Cramps

Some research suggests that relaxation techniques may be beneficial for menstrual cramps, but definite conclusions can't be reached because of the small number of participants in the studies and the poor quality of some of the research.

Nausea

An evaluation of the research evidence concluded that some relaxation techniques, including guided imagery and progressive muscle relaxation, are likely to be effective in relieving nausea caused by cancer chemotherapy when used in combination with antinausea drugs.

Nightmares

Some studies have indicated that relaxation exercises may be an effective approach for nightmares of unknown cause and those associated with posttraumatic stress disorder (PTSD). However, an assessment of many studies concluded that relaxation is less helpful than more extensive forms of treatment (psychotherapy or medication).

Pain

Evaluations of the research evidence have found promising but not conclusive evidence that guided imagery may help relieve some musculoskeletal pain (pain involving the bones or muscles) and other types of pain.

An analysis of data on hospitalized cancer patients showed that those who received integrative medicine therapies, such as guided imagery, and relaxation response training, during their hospitalization had reductions in both pain and anxiety.

Pain In Children And Adolescents

A 2014 evaluation of the scientific evidence found that psychological therapies, which may include relaxation techniques as well as other approaches such as CBT, can reduce pain in children and adolescents with chronic headaches or other types of chronic pain. The evidence is particularly promising for headaches: the effect on pain may last for several months after treatment, and the therapies also help to reduce anxiety.

Posttraumatic Stress Disorder

Studies of biofeedback and other relaxation techniques for PTSD have had inconsistent results.

Rheumatoid Arthritis (RA)

There's limited evidence that biofeedback or other relaxation techniques might be valuable additions to treatment programs for RA.

Ringing In The Ears (Tinnitus)

Only a few studies have evaluated relaxation techniques for ringing in the ears. The limited evidence from these studies suggests that relaxation techniques might be useful, especially in reducing the intrusiveness of the problem.

Smoking Cessation

- Limited evidence suggests that guided imagery may be a valuable tool for people who are working to quit smoking.
- In a study that compared the two techniques, autogenic training was found to be less effective than CBT as a quit smoking aid. However, this study involved patients in an alcohol detoxification program, so its results may not be applicable to other people.

- Preliminary research suggests that a guided relaxation routine might help reduce cigarette cravings.

Temporomandibular Joint Dysfunction (TMD)

Problems with the temporomandibular joint (the joint that connects the jaw to the side of the head) can cause pain and difficulty moving the jaw. A few studies have shown that programs that include relaxation techniques may help relieve symptoms of TMD.

What The Science Says About The Safety And Side Effects Of Relaxation Techniques

- Relaxation techniques are generally considered safe for healthy people. However, occasionally, people report negative experiences such as increased anxiety, intrusive thoughts, or fear of losing control.
- There have been rare reports that certain relaxation techniques might cause or worsen symptoms in people with epilepsy or certain psychiatric conditions, or with a history of abuse or trauma. People with heart disease should talk to their healthcare provider before doing progressive muscle relaxation.

Chapter 27

Meditation

What Is Meditation?

Meditation is a mind and body practice that has a long history of use for increasing calmness and physical relaxation, improving psychological balance, coping with illness, and enhancing overall health and well-being. Mind and body practices focus on the interactions among the brain, mind, body, and behavior.

There are many types of meditation, but most have four elements in common: a quiet location with as few distractions as possible; a specific, comfortable posture (sitting, lying down, walking, or in other positions); a focus of attention (a specially chosen word or set of words, an object, or the sensations of the breath); and an open attitude (letting distractions come and go naturally without judging them).

Meditation has been used for centuries to increase calmness and physical relaxation, improve psychological balance, cope with illness, and enhance overall health and well-being. Meditation can take a variety of forms: mantra meditation, relaxation response, mindfulness meditation, Transcendental Meditation, and Zen Buddhist meditation, among others. Yoga and Tai chi also incorporate meditative components. Meditation practices are often rooted in spiritual practices, but many people practice meditation outside of a religious context.

(Source: "Exploring The Power Of Meditation," National Center for Complementary and Integrative Health (NCCIH).)

About This Chapter: Text beginning with the heading "What Is Meditation?" is excerpted from "Meditation: In Depth," National Center for Complementary and Integrative Health (NCCIH), April 2016; Text under the heading "Eight Things To Know About Meditation For Health" is excerpted from "8 Things To Know About Meditation For Health," National Center for Complementary and Integrative Health (NCCIH), January 30, 2018.

What The Science Says About The Effectiveness Of Meditation

Many studies have investigated meditation for different conditions, and there's evidence that it may reduce blood pressure as well as symptoms of irritable bowel syndrome (IBS) and flare-ups in people who have had ulcerative colitis (UC). It may ease symptoms of anxiety and depression, and may help people with insomnia.

Pain

- Research about meditation's ability to reduce pain has produced mixed results. However, in some studies scientists suggest that meditation activates certain areas of the brain in response to pain.
- A small study funded in part by the National Center for Complementary and Integrative Health (NCCIH) found that mindfulness meditation does help to control pain and doesn't use the brain's naturally occurring opiates to do so. This suggests that combining mindfulness with pain medications and other approaches that rely on the brain's opioid activity may be particularly effective for reducing pain.

For High Blood Pressure

- Results of a NCCIH funded trial involving 298 university students suggest that practicing transcendental meditation (TM) may lower the blood pressure of people at increased risk of developing high blood pressure.
- The findings also suggested that practicing meditation can help with psychological distress, anxiety, depression, anger/hostility, and coping ability.
- A literature review and scientific statement from the American Heart Association (AHA) suggest that evidence supports the use of TM to lower blood pressure. However, the review indicates that it's uncertain whether TM is truly superior to other meditation techniques in terms of blood-pressure lowering because there are few head to head studies.

For Irritable Bowel Syndrome (IBS)

- The few studies that have looked at mindfulness meditation training for irritable bowel syndrome found no clear effects, the American College of Gastroenterology (ACG) stated in a report. But the researchers noted that given the limited number of studies, they can't be sure that IBS doesn't help.

- Results of another NCCIH funded trial that enrolled 75 women suggest that practicing mindfulness meditation for 8 weeks reduces the severity of IBS symptoms.
- Another review concluded that mindfulness training improved IBS patients' pain and quality of life but not their depression or anxiety. The amount of improvement was small.

For Smoking Cessation

- The results of 13 studies of mindfulness-based interventions for stopping smoking had promising results regarding craving, smoking cessation, and relapse prevention, a research review found. However, the studies had many limitations.
- Findings from a review suggest that meditation based therapies may help people quit smoking; however, the small number of available studies is insufficient to determine rigorously if meditation is effective for this.
- A trial comparing mindfulness training with a standard behavioral smoking cessation treatment found that individuals who received mindfulness training showed a greater rate of reduction in cigarette use immediately after treatment and at 17-week follow-up.
- Results of a brain imaging study suggest that mindful attention reduced the craving to smoke, and also that it reduced activity in a craving related region of the brain.
- However, in a second brain imaging study, researchers observed that a 2-week course of meditation (5 hours total) significantly reduced smoking, compared with relaxation training, and that it increased activity in brain areas associated with craving.

Other Conditions

- Guidelines from the American College of Chest Physicians (ACCP) published in 2013 suggest that MBSR and meditation may help to reduce stress, anxiety, pain, and depression while enhancing mood and self-esteem in people with lung cancer.
- Clinical practice guidelines issued in 2014 by the Society for Integrative Oncology (SIO) recommend meditation as supportive care to reduce stress, anxiety, depression, and fatigue in patients treated for breast cancer. The serum insulin concentration (SIC) also recommends its use to improve quality of life in these people.
- Meditation based programs may be helpful in reducing common menopausal symptoms, including the frequency and intensity of hot flashes, sleep and mood disturbances, stress, and muscle and joint pain. However, differences in study designs mean that no firm conclusions can be drawn.

- Because only a few studies have been conducted on the effects of meditation for attention deficit hyperactivity disorder (ADHD), there isn't sufficient evidence to support its use for this condition.
- A research review suggested that mind and body practices, including meditation, reduce chemical identifiers of inflammation and show promise in helping to regulate the immune system.

Meditation And The Brain

Some research suggests that meditation may physically change the brain and body and could potentially help to improve many health problems and promote healthy behaviors.

- A review of three studies suggests that meditation may slow, stall, or even reverse changes that take place in the brain due to normal aging.
- Results from a NCCIH funded study suggest that meditation can affect activity in the amygdala (a part of the brain involved in processing emotions), and that different types of meditation can affect the amygdala differently even when the person is not meditating.
- Research about meditation's ability to reduce pain has produced mixed results. However, in some studies scientists suggest that meditation activates certain areas of the brain in response to pain.

What The Science Says About Safety And Side Effects Of Meditation

- Meditation is generally considered to be safe for healthy people.
- People with physical limitations may not be able to participate in certain meditative practices involving movement. People with physical health conditions should speak with their healthcare providers before starting a meditative practice, and make their meditation instructor aware of their condition.
- There have been rare reports that meditation could cause or worsen symptoms in people with certain psychiatric problems like anxiety and depression. People with existing mental health conditions should speak with their healthcare providers before starting a meditative practice, and make their meditation instructor aware of their condition.

Meditation is a mind and body practice that has a long history of use for increasing calmness and physical relaxation, improving psychological balance, coping with illness, and enhancing overall health and well-being. Many studies have been conducted to look at how meditation may be helpful for a variety of conditions, such as high blood pressure, certain psychological disorders, and pain. A number of studies also have helped researchers learn how meditation might work and how it affects the brain.

Eight Things To Know About Meditation For Health

Here are eight things to know about what the science says about meditation for health:

1. For people who suffer from cancer symptoms and treatment side effects, mind-body therapies, such as meditation, have been shown to help relieve anxiety, stress, fatigue, and general mood and sleep disturbances, thus improving their quality of life. Evidence-based clinical practice guidelines from the Society for Integrative Oncology (SIO) recommend meditation, as well as other mind-body modalities, as part of a multidisciplinary approach to reduce anxiety, mood disturbance, chronic pain, and improve quality of life.
2. There is some evidence that meditation may reduce blood pressure. A literature review and scientific statement from the American Heart Association (AHA) suggests that evidence supports the use of transcendental meditation as an adjunct or complementary therapy along with standard treatment to lower blood pressure.
3. A growing body of evidence suggests that meditation-based programs may be helpful in reducing common menopausal symptoms. A review of scientific literature found that yoga, tai chi, and meditation-based programs may be helpful in reducing common menopausal symptoms including the frequency and intensity of hot flashes, sleep and mood disturbances, stress, and muscle and joint pain.
4. There is moderate evidence that meditation improves symptoms of anxiety. A review of the literature found that mindfulness meditation programs had moderate evidence of improved anxiety, depression, and pain, and low evidence of improved stress/distress and mental health-related quality of life.
5. Some studies suggest that mindfulness meditation helps people with irritable bowel syndrome (IBS), but there's not enough evidence to draw firm conclusions. A review of the scientific literature concluded that mindfulness training improved IBS patients' pain and quality of life but not their depression or anxiety; however, the amount of improvement was small.

6. Overall, there is not enough evidence to know whether mind-body practices are as effective as other treatments to help people quit smoking. To date, there have only been a few studies on mindfulness-based therapies to aid in smoking cessation.
7. There isn't enough evidence to support the use of meditation for attention deficit hyperactivity disorder (ADHD). According to a review of the science, because of the small number of studies conducted on meditation for ADHD, no conclusions could be drawn about its effectiveness for this condition.
8. Meditation is generally considered to be safe for healthy people. However, people with physical limitations may not be able to participate in certain meditative practices involving movement.

Chapter 28

Hypnotherapy

That time you were totally absorbed, whether you were sinking every jumpshot or flying around Hogwarts? Well, you just might have been under hypnosis. Researchers believe that super-focused trance-like states can be harnessed to treat medical problems—to reduce pain or control neuromuscular disorders, for instance.

"Hypnosis is the oldest Western conception of a psychotherapy," said National Institute of Health (NIH) grantee Dr. David Spiegel in a National Center for Complementary and Integrative Health (NCCIH) Integrative Medicine Research Lecture. "It's the first time a talking interaction was thought to have therapeutic potential. It's useful as a model system for understanding how brain-body interactions work."

Spiegel is medical director of the Center for Integrative Medicine at Stanford University School of Medicine. His research—with funding over the years from National Institutes of Health (NIH), National Cancer Institute (NCI), National Institute of Mental Health (NIMH) and NCCIH—spans four decades in such areas as psycho-oncology, stress and health, pain control and clinical applications of hypnosis.

About This Chapter: Text in this chapter begins with excerpts from "How Can Hypnosis Treat Medical Problems?" National Institutes of Health (NIH), June 19, 2015; Text under the heading "How Can Hypnosis Treat Medical Problems?" is excerpted from "Hypnosis," National Center for Complementary and Integrative Health (NCCIH), September 24, 2017; Text under the heading "Hypnotherapy And Irritable Bowel Syndrome (IBS)" is excerpted from "6 Tips: IBS And Complementary Health Practices," National Center for Complementary and Integrative Health (NCCIH), September 24, 2015; Text under the heading "Hypnotherapy And Smoking Cessation" is excerpted from "Complementary Health Approaches For Smoking Cessation: What The Science Says," National Center for Complementary and Integrative Health (NCCIH), November 13, 2017.

History Of Hypnosis

Viennese physician Franz Anton Mesmer founded the field. In the 18th century, "he theorized that magnetic fields flow through the body. When people got sick, something went wrong with their magnetic fields. [Mesmer believed] if he put his magnetic field next to their magnetic field, theirs would get better." Mesmer moved to France, where his practice flourished. Not really surprising, Spiegel said. Compare hypnosis with what French doctors were using back then—bloodletting. Patients under the care of French physicians were more prone to die.

Mesmer's success did not endear him to the French medical establishment, which begged King Louis to investigate the Viennese doctor. A panel that included Benjamin Franklin and "pain-control expert" Dr. Joseph-Ignace Guillotin, inventor of the execution device that bears his name, concluded Mesmer's method was "nothing but heated imagination."

That episode ended Mesmer's career and recorded perhaps the first doubt about trances as medicine. It did not prevent further pursuit of hypnosis' potential healing powers nor further skepticism. Hypnosis, Spiegel quipped, "has been something like the oldest profession—everybody's interested in it, but no one wants to be seen in public with it. It was at the foundation of many very important movements, including psychoanalysis."

Sigmund Freud began psychoanalysis by using hypnosis as "a royal road to the unconscious," Spiegel said. When Freud found some patients formed irrational feelings for their physicians during hypnosis, he stopped the practice. Instead of entering trance-like states, patients were urged to free associate. At the end of his career, however, Freud returned to an interest in hypnosis.

You Are Not Getting Very Sleepy

Defining hypnosis as a "state of aroused, attentive, focused concentration with diminished peripheral awareness," Spiegel also refuted a common misconception. "You don't go to sleep," he said. "Hypnosis is not sleep. It's a narrowing of the focus of attention. Hypnosis is to consciousness what a telephoto lens is to a camera: What you see you see with great detail, but you're less aware of the context."

So, can hypnosis make folks flap their arms and squawk like a chicken? No, usually not. Some vulnerability does come with the practice, though. "People in hypnosis are less likely to critically judge what you say to them," noted Spiegel, explaining suggestibility. "You've got to be careful what you say to them, because they're less likely to correct your mistakes. It makes people nervous, because we are all social creatures. We all respond to social cues and sometimes we do so irrationally. Hypnosis is an example of how much we can allow input from other people—even people we don't know very well—to control our perception, judgment and behavior."

In The Zone?

We use hypnotic-like states in normal activities, Spiegel said. "Self-hypnosis is what people do when they want to enhance performance." Top athletes commonly describe their training techniques for competing at their highest levels as involving intensely focused imagination. They visualize their best performance to the exclusion of all else around them. Spiegel said that type of laser-focused attention is a form of self-hypnosis.

"People who are more highly hypnotizable have more self-altering states of attention—total absorption—in everyday life all the time," Spiegel noted. "They get lost in a sunset or a movie or reading a novel."

Studies indicate that hypnotizability cannot be taught. In fact, Spiegel said, it's a more stable trait over the lifespan than Intelligence quotient (IQ). Researchers estimate that about one-third of people cannot be hypnotized, while 15 percent of the population is considered highly hypnotizable. The rest of us have varying degrees of hypnotizability that we can be trained to use.

In terms of neurophysiology, Spiegel said researchers see brain differences between people who are high and low in hypnotizability. The brain's anterior cingulate cortex (ACC) region—where tasks such as attention, monitoring and pain management are located—seems to play a significant role in hypnotic experience.

Scientists have collected "data showing how if you change how distressing pain is—not the sensation itself, but how much it bothers you—then you reduce activity in the [ACC] as well," he explained.

Highly hypnotizable individuals have more functional connectivity—a functional magnetic resonance imaging (fMRI) term for neurons that fire together—between the dorsal ACC and portions of the executive control network in the dorsolateral prefrontal cortex, Spiegel pointed out. This means that paying attention and carrying out a task are highly coordinated among high hypnotizables, he said.

Researchers conducted brain scans of study participants while they were under hypnosis. Scientists examined which brain regions turn on and off and which areas work together. These studies helped clarify how dissociation occurs, Spiegel said.

"When you're engaged in hypnosis, you're not ruminating about yourself," he noted. "People will engage in hypnotic experiences and they often won't remember what they did. We think it has to do with an inverse relationship between being hypnotized and functioning of the [brain's] default mode network. We're beginning to understand what goes on in the brain when people enter these altered states."

Change Your Mind

Spiegel showed videos of some of his clinical work. In one clip, a patient with Parkinson disease who experienced near-constant involuntary tremors in his hand was able, under self-hypnosis, to rest his hand. He imagined himself in his happy place—Hawaii, in this case—and the tremors stopped.

Spiegel shared results from some of his group's other studies:

- One out of four patients under hypnosis can permanently quit smoking.
- Self-hypnotized metastatic breast cancer patients were able to cut their pain levels in half.
- Children taught to imagine themselves elsewhere better tolerated a painful invasive medical exam; procedure time was reduced by 17 minutes.

"In hypnosis, you actually use words to transform perception," Spiegel concluded. "So some of our ability to manipulate experience is not just from speech and motor activity but also from the ability to control our own perceptual processes. We have an amazing ability in our brain to alter not just how we react to perception but also what it is that we perceive. If you think it is taking away control, it isn't. Hypnosis is teaching people control."

How Can Hypnosis Treat Medical Problems?

Hypnosis (also called hypnotherapy) has been studied for a number of conditions, including state anxiety (e.g., before medical procedures or surgeries), headaches, smoking cessation, pain control, hot flashes in breast cancer survivors, and irritable bowel syndrome.

Hypnotherapy And Irritable Bowel Syndrome (IBS)

This practice involves the power of suggestion by a trained hypnotist or hypnotherapist during a state of deep relaxation, and is the most widely used mind and body intervention for IBS. According to reviews of the scientific literature, hypnotherapy may be a helpful treatment for managing IBS symptoms. Several studies of hypnotherapy for IBS have shown substantial long-term improvement of gastrointestinal symptoms as well as anxiety, depression, disability, and quality of life.

Hypnotherapy And Smoking Cessation

There is some evidence to suggest that hypnotherapy may improve smoking cessation, but data are not definitive.

What Does The Research Show?

- A 2014 randomized controlled trial of 164 patients hospitalized with cardiac or pulmonary illness compared the efficacy of hypnotherapy alone, as well as hypnotherapy with nicotine replacement therapy, to conventional nicotine replacement therapy alone. The study found that hypnotherapy patients were more likely than nicotine replacement therapy patients to be nonsmokers at 12 weeks and 26 weeks after hospitalization.
- A 2010 Cochrane review of eleven studies compared hypnotherapy with 18 different control interventions. The authors found that hypnotherapy did not have a greater effect on 6-month quit rates than other interventions or no treatment. They concluded that there is not enough evidence to show whether hypnotherapy could be as effective as counseling treatment.
- A 2012 meta-analysis of randomized controlled trials found that acupuncture, hypnotherapy, and aversive smoking increased smoking abstinence, but the patient population in the analysis was small and reports of smoking cessation were not validated by biochemical means.

Safety Considerations Of Hypnotherapy

Hypnosis is considered safe when performed by a health professional trained in hypnotherapy.

Self-hypnosis also appears to be safe for most people. There are no reported cases of injury resulting from self hypnosis.

Chapter 29

Aromatherapy

What Is Aromatherapy?

Aromatherapy is the use of essential oils from plants to support and balance the mind, body, and spirit. It is used by patients mainly as a form of supportive care that may improve quality of life and reduce stress, anxiety, and nausea, and vomiting caused by chemotherapy. Aromatherapy may be combined with other complementary treatments like massage therapy, and acupuncture, as well as with standard treatments, for symptom management.

Essential oils (also known as volatile oils) are the basic materials of aromatherapy. They represent the fragrant essences found in many plants. These essences are made in special plant cells, often under the surface of leaves, bark, or peel, using energy from the sun and elements from the air, soil, and water. If the plant is crushed, the essence and its unique fragrance are released.

When essences are extracted from plants, they become essential oils. They may be distilled with steam and/or water, or mechanically pressed. Essential oils that are made by processes that modify their chemistry are not considered true essential oils.

There are many essential oils used in aromatherapy, including those from Roman chamomile, geranium, lavender, tea tree, lemon, ginger, cedarwood, and bergamot. Each plant's essential oil has a different chemical composition that affects how it smells, how it is absorbed, and how it is used by the body. Even the essential oils from varieties of the same plant species may have chemical compositions different from each other. The same applies to plants that are grown or harvested in different ways or locations.

About This Chapter: This chapter includes text excerpted from "Aromatherapy And Essential Oils (PDQ®)—Patient Version," National Cancer Institute (NCI), June 9, 2017.

Essential oils are very concentrated. For example, it takes about 220 lbs of lavender flowers to make about 1 pound of essential oil. Essential oils are volatile, evaporating quickly when they are exposed to open air.

What Is The History Of The Discovery And Use Of Aromatherapy As A Complementary And Alternative Treatment?

Fragrant plants have been used in healing practices for thousands of years across many cultures, including ancient China, India, and Egypt. Ways to extract essential oils from plants were first discovered during the Middle Ages.

Smelling And Your Health

Your sense of smell enriches your experience of the world around you. Different scents can change your mood, transport you back to a distant memory, and may even help you bond with loved ones. Your ability to smell also plays a key role in your health. If your ability to smell declines, it can affect your diet and nutrition, physical well-being, and everyday safety.

Because smell information is sent to different parts of the brain, odors can influence many aspects of our lives, such as memory, mood, and emotion. For thousands of years, fragrant plants have been used in healing practices across many cultures, including ancient China, India, and Egypt. Aromatherapy, for example, aims to use essential oils from flowers, herbs, or trees to improve physical and emotional well-being.

(Source: "What Your Nose Knows—Sense Of Smell And Your Health," NIH News in Health, *National Institutes of Health (NIH).)*

The history of modern aromatherapy began in the early 20th century, when French chemist Rene Gattefosse coined the term *aromatherapy* and studied the effects of essential oils on many kinds of diseases. In the 1980s and 1990s, aromatherapy was rediscovered in Western countries as interest in complementary and alternative medicine (CAM) began to grow.

What Is The Theory Behind The Claim That Aromatherapy Is Useful In Treating Cancer?

Aromatherapy is rarely suggested as a treatment for cancer, but rather as a form of supportive care to manage symptoms of cancer or side effects of cancer treatment. There are different theories about how aromatherapy and essential oils work. A leading theory is that smell receptors in the nose may respond to the smells of essential oils by sending chemical messages along nerve pathways to the brain's limbic system, which affects moods, and emotions. Imaging studies in humans help show the effects of smells on the limbic system and its emotional pathways.

How Is Aromatherapy Administered?

Aromatherapy is used in various ways. Examples include:

- Indirect inhalation (patient breathes in an essential oil by using a room diffuser or placing drops nearby).
- Direct inhalation (patient breathes in an essential oil by using an individual inhaler with drops floated on top of hot water) to treat a sinus headache.
- Aromatherapy massage (massaging of one or more essential oils, diluted in a carrier oil, into the skin).
- Applying essential oils to the skin by combining them with bath salts, lotions, or dressings.
- Aromatherapy is rarely taken by mouth.

There are some essential oils commonly chosen to treat specific conditions. However, the types of oils used and the ways they are combined may vary, depending on the experience and training of the aromatherapist. This lack of standard methods has led to some conflicting research on the effects of aromatherapy.

Have Any Preclinical (Laboratory Or Animal) Studies Been Conducted Using Aromatherapy?

Many studies of essential oils have found that they have antibacterial effects when applied to the skin. Some essential oils have antiviral activity against the herpes simplex virus. Others have antifungal activity against certain vaginal and oropharyngeal fungal infections. In addition, studies in rats have shown that different essential oils can be calming or energizing. When rats were exposed to certain fragrances under stressful conditions, their behavior and immune responses were improved.

One study showed that after essential oils were inhaled, markers of the fragrance compounds were found in the bloodstream, suggesting that aromatherapy affects the body directly like a drug, in addition to indirectly through the central nervous system (CNS).

Have Any Clinical Trials (Research Studies With People) Of Aromatherapy Been Conducted?

Clinical trials of aromatherapy have mainly studied its use in the treatment of nausea and vomiting caused by chemotherapy, stress, anxiety, and other health related conditions in seriously ill patients. Several clinical trials of aromatherapy in patients with cancer have been published with mixed results.

A few early studies have shown that aromatherapy may improve quality of life in patients with cancer. Some patients receiving aromatherapy have reported improvement in symptoms such as nausea, or pain, and have lower blood pressure, pulse, and respiratory rates. Studies of aromatherapy massage have had mixed results, with some studies reporting improvement in mood, anxiety, pain, and constipation and other studies reporting no effect.

A study of inhaled bergamot essential oil in children and adolescents receiving stem cell transplants reported an increase in anxiety and nausea and no effect on pain. Parents receiving the aromatherapy and parents receiving the placebo both showed less anxiety after their children's transplants. In a study of adult patients receiving stem cell transplants, tasting or sniffing sliced oranges was more effective at reducing nausea, retching, and coughing than inhaling an orange essential oil.

A small study of tea tree essential oil as a topical treatment to clear antibiotic resistant Methicillin resistant Staphylococcus aureus (MRSA) bacteria from the skin of hospital patients found that it was as effective as the standard treatment. Antibacterial essential oils have been studied to lessen odor in necrotic ulcers.

No studies in scientific or medical literature discuss aromatherapy as a treatment for cancer specifically.

Have Any Side Effects Or Risks Been Reported From Aromatherapy?

Safety testing on essential oils shows very few side effects or risks when they are used as directed. Some essential oils have been approved as ingredients in food and are classified as GRAS (generally recognized as safe) by the U.S. Food and Drug Administration (FDA), within specific limits. Swallowing large amounts of essential oils is not recommended.

Allergic reactions and skin irritation may occur in aromatherapists or in patients, especially when essential oils are in contact with the skin for long periods of time. Sun sensitivity may develop when citrus or other essential oils are applied to the skin before sun exposure.

Lavender and tea tree essential oils have been found to have some hormone like effects. They have effects similar to estrogen (female sex hormone) and also block or decrease the effect of androgens (male sex hormones). Applying lavender and tea tree essential oils to the skin over a long-period of time has been linked in one study to breast enlargement in boys who have not yet reached puberty. It is recommended that patients with tumors that need estrogen to grow avoid using lavender and tea tree essential oils.

Is Aromatherapy Approved By The U.S. Food And Drug Administration (FDA) For Use As A Cancer Treatment In The United States?

Aromatherapy products do not need approval by the FDA because no specific claims are made for the treatment of cancer or other diseases.

Aromatherapy is not regulated by state law, and there is no licensing required to practice aromatherapy in the United States. Professionals often combine aromatherapy training with another field in which they are licensed, for example, massage therapy, registered nursing, acupuncture, or naturopathy. Some aromatherapy courses for healthcare providers offer medical credit hours and include conducting research and measuring results.

Chapter 30

Guided Imagery

What Is Visualization/Guided Imagery?[1]

Imagery is a nonphysiological (cognitive) relaxation technique that can be used to ease stress and promote an overall sense of well-being. Imagery focuses on increasing cognitive, emotional, and physical control by changing the focus of an individual's thoughts. We all have daydreamed about pleasant things that have distracted us and made us feel better. Imagery uses much the same process but encourages positive adaptive "dreaming" that distracts and relaxes the individual. Imagery is highly effective for depression and anxiety, as well as specific situations that require clarity, focus, distraction, or feelings of mastery. The following are examples:

Table 30.1. Imagery

Topic	Focused Topic	Image	Outcome
Depression	Negative Self-worth	Images of success or past situations of success; images of a pleasant past experience	Increased self-confidence; reduced negative thoughts; distraction from negative mood
Anxiety/Worry	Public Speaking	Image of speech that goes well; image of something funny	Reduced negative focus, distraction, increased positive expectations

About This Chapter: This chapter includes text excerpted from documents published by two public domain sources. Text under the headings marked 1 are excerpted from "A Therapist's Guide To Brief Cognitive Behavioral Therapy," U.S. Department of Veterans Affairs (VA), January 30, 2010. Reviewed January 2018; Text under heading marked 2 is excerpted from "Visualization/Guided Imagery," U.S. Department of Veterans Affairs (VA), July 2013. Reviewed January 2018.

Table 30.1. Continued

Topic	Focused Topic	Image	Outcome
Medical Anxiety	Fear of Procedure (e.g., needles)	Relaxation; peacefulness; pain-free environment	Less tension, reduced anxiety, toleration of procedure with less distress
Sports Performance	Focused efforts during golf game	Envisioning the desired shot; positive words of advice	Increased focus, self-confidence, thinking

How Guided Imagery Works[1]

Research has shown that the mind can actually affect how the body functions. It seems the body may not know the difference between an actual event and a thought. Guided imagery uses the power of the brain—images and the perception that you are either somewhere else or in a different state of mind—to increase pleasant experiences and performance to promote wellness and health. On the flip side, imagery helps to reduce stress tension and anxiety by changing thoughts and emotions or through distraction.

Imagery is commonly referred to as guided imagery. Guided imagery refers to a process whereby you facilitate or guide the initial images the patient uses. The following section describes how you can guide the patient into the effective use of imagery for relaxation or performance improvement.

Step 1: Introduce imagery.

Introduce imagery to the patient, pointing out the power of the brain or thoughts and how images, when accessed correctly, can actually change physical and emotional states.

Step 2: Identify the desired outcomes, such as decreased anxiety, increased focus, distraction.

Step 3: Develop an image or scene.

Work with the patient on the third step to identify a situation, either in the past or a place he/she would like to be, that both you and the patient feel might benefit or produce the desired outcome. Sample imagery scripts are provided below and can be used if the patient has difficulty creating a personal situation. Selection of a powerful image is critical to the success of this technique. Selection of an image that the patient is able to fully embrace increases the odds of treatment success. Selection of a "weak" image (e.g., not viewed as important by the patient or unable to be fully visualized) will likely lead to treatment failure.

Step 4: Increase vividness of the image.

To ensure that patients find a "strong" image, ask them to explore as many senses as possible to increase vividness of the image. For example, when imagining a glass of lemonade, imagine holding a glass that feels icy and cold, visualize the color of the lemonade, think of the fresh citrus smell, and finally think of how the lemonade tastes. This is an example of imagery that uses multiple senses and increases vividness of the image. Increasing vividness is largely a matter of increasing the details the patient experiences. The more details described by the patient, the more powerful the technique.

Step 5: Ask the patient if he or she notices any changes after the imagery exercise.

Step 6: Repeat the imagery exercise until the patient reports skill understanding and benefit.

Step 7: Ask the patient to identify situations when imagery might be appropriate. Expand upon the patient's responses by adding other situations (e.g., how the technique can be used).

Other tips for imagery:

1. Pair up imagery with deep-breathing exercises.
2. Ask patient to close eyes during the exercise to increase vividness.
3. Interject during the imagery experience aspects that you feel might benefit the patient. For example, a patient might use the beach image; and you might ask how the sun feels on the skin, whether he or she hears anything, or what else he or she sees.
4. Help the patient focus on aspects of the image that will guide him/her towards the goal. Help the patient to avoid too many unnecessary details that might distract from the goal.
5. Point out that imagery is a portable skill that the patient can use in a variety of situations and completely without notice of others.
6. Avoid imagery with psychotic patients, who might confuse reality with images.

Script 1: Generic Example[1]

Once your whole body feels relaxed, travel to your favorite place, it can be any time period or any place. This place is calm and safe—there are no worries here—look around this place. What do you see? Do you hear the sounds around you? What are some of the sounds you hear in this place you are imagining? How does this special place smell? Walk around a little, and take in all the wonderful sights. Feel the air around you and relax.... The air is fresh, and it's easy to breathe here. Pay attention to how your body feels. Say to yourself, "I am totally relaxed... without worries... all the tension has drained away from my body." Take a moment to fully experience your favorite place. Notice the sounds, the sights, smells, and how it feels to be in this very special place. Remember that you can visit this place as often as you want and that it is wonderful. Say to yourself, "I am relaxed here... this place is special and makes me feel at peace." When you are done with your visit to this special place, open your eyes and stay in your comfortable position. Continue to breathe smoothly, in a relaxed and rhythmic fashion. Take as long as you want to enjoy and relax. Feel at ease knowing your special place is always available to you, and find that you feel relaxed, even after you leave.

Script 2: The Beach[1]

Imagine yourself walking down a sandy beach. The sand is white and warm between your toes. You are looking out over the calm, blue water. The waves are gently lapping at the shore. You feel the pleasant warmth of the sun on your skin... it's a perfectly comfortable temperature outside. Breathe in deeply. There is a gentle breeze, and the sun is shining. Big, cotton-like clouds drift by as you hear seagulls in the distance. You taste traces of salt on your lips. You are completely relaxed... there are no worries on this beach. There is nothing to distract you from feeling tranquil. Worries drift away. Notice the sounds, sights, smells, and how it feels to be in this very special place.

Feel the sand under your feet... you decide to stretch out on the warm, fine, white sand... breathe deeply... feel the warm air. Your body is completely relaxed, and you have an overall feeling of warmth and comfort. You look up at the clouds pass by slowly across the beautiful blue sky. You are feeling rejuvenated and completely at peace. Remember that you can visit this place as often as you want and that it is wonderful. Say to yourself, "I am relaxed here... this place is special and makes me feel peaceful and content." When you are done with your visit, open your eyes and stay in your comfortable position. Continue to breathe smoothly, in a relaxed and rhythmic fashion; take as long as you want to enjoy and relax. You feel at ease knowing your special place is always available to you, and you find that you feel relaxed even after you leave.

Script 3: The Private Garden[2]

Close your eyes. Allow yourself to get comfortable... begin with a few slow deep breaths in through your nose and out through your mouth, letting your body get relaxed. Let the chair fully support your body as you continue to breath and relax.

Now, use your imagination to picture yourself walking slowly along a path. It's a pleasant path, any kind that you wish. It's a beautiful day, and you feel relaxed and happy. You can feel the warmth and energy of the sunlight on your skin... soon you come to a gate. You know this gate leads to a special place where you feel welcomed, safe, and comfortable. Push the gate open and allow yourself to enter your very own private garden.

Your garden is filled with your favorite things. Whatever is pleasing to you can be found in this place. Perhaps there are flowers, trees, animals, birds, water, or even music. Look around and notice what is in your garden... see all the colors and objects that are in this place. Notice how beautiful they are... look at the various shapes and see how varied they are... look at the ground, look at the sky, and see where they meet... your garden is calm and tranquil. Everything peacefully coexists in the garden... as you are looking, become aware of how things might feel in this private place of yours. Begin to explore this place with your sense of touch. Perhaps some things are soft and warm, and others are smooth and cool. Simply spend some time exploring, using your sense of touch as you continue to feel at peace and comfortable... notice what the air feels like; is it cool or warm?... is there a breeze or is it still?... take the time to feel the peace and serenity in this private place... as you continue to explore your garden by seeing and feeling, become aware of the sounds that you hear in your garden... the sounds in your garden are pleasing to the ear and very comforting. Perhaps it is quiet in your garden, or maybe there are a number of sounds. Some of the sounds may be very soft, while others may be louder. Relax and listen for a while and see if you can identify the different sounds in your garden... as you're listening to the sounds in your garden, become aware of what smells you might smell. Take a deep breath in, and notice the fragrances that are present. Some of them may be familiar, while others may be unfamiliar. The fragrances are pleasant and soothing... take your time and enjoy your visit to the garden, using it in whatever way that you wish. Spend the time that is necessary for you to rejuvenate and to care for yourself.

When you are ready to leave, slowly walk back towards the gate of your garden. You have enjoyed your visit to the garden and feel relaxed and content. This good feeling will remain with you throughout the day. Push the gate open and return to the path that led you to the garden. As you make your way back up the path to the here and now, remember that you can use your imagination to return to your private garden at any time you wish. Visit your garden any time you would like to relax, to be comforted, or just to enjoy its beauty... you are now ready to resume your day. Stretch gently and open your eyes, feeling refreshed and alert.

Other Guided Imagery Scene Suggestions[1]

- A mountain scene where you feel calm and relaxed as you look out over the valley. Just you and the vegetation and you dip your feet into a cool mountain stream; and let your foot rest on a big, slippery stone as the sunshine warms you and the wind blows through the trees.
- Advanced scenarios developed with assistance of patient (family, past experiences, etc.).

Chapter 31

Spirituality

Studies have shown that religious and spiritual values are important to Americans. Most Americans say that they believe in God and that their religious beliefs affect how they live their lives. However, people have different ideas about life after death, belief in miracles, and other religious beliefs. Such beliefs may be based on gender, education, and ethnic background.

Many patients rely on spiritual or religious beliefs and practices to help them cope with their disease. This is called spiritual coping. Many caregivers also rely on spiritual coping. Each person may have different spiritual needs, depending on cultural and religious traditions. For some seriously ill patients, spiritual well-being may affect how much anxiety they feel about death. For others, it may affect what they decide about end-of-life treatments. Some patients and their family caregivers may want doctors to talk about spiritual concerns, but may feel unsure about how to bring up the subject.

Some studies show that doctors' support of spiritual well-being in very ill patients helps improve their quality of life. Healthcare providers who treat patients coping with cancer are looking at new ways to help them with religious and spiritual concerns. Doctors may ask patients which spiritual issues are important to them during treatment as well as near the end of life. When patients with advanced cancer receive spiritual support from the medical team, they may be more likely to choose hospice care and less aggressive treatment at the end of life.

About This Chapter: Text in this chapter begins with excerpts from "Spirituality in Cancer Care (PDQ®)—Patient Version," National Cancer Institute (NCI), May 18, 2015; Text under the heading "Three Types of Spirituality" is excerpted from "Three Types of Spirituality," U.S. Department of Veterans Affairs (VA), January 12, 2016.

Spirituality And Religion May Have Different Meanings

The terms spirituality and religion are often used in place of each other, but for many people they have different meanings. Religion may be defined as a specific set of beliefs and practices, usually within an organized group. Spirituality may be defined as an individual's sense of peace, purpose, and connection to others, and beliefs about the meaning of life. Spirituality may be found and expressed through an organized religion or in other ways. Patients may think of themselves as spiritual or religious or both.

What Spirituality Means

Spirituality is a personal experience with many definitions. Spirituality might be defined as "an inner belief system providing an individual with meaning and purpose in life, a sense of the sacredness of life, and a vision for the betterment of the world." Other definitions emphasize "a connection to that which transcends the self." The connection might be to God, a higher power, a universal energy, the sacred, or to nature. Researchers in the field of spirituality have suggested three useful dimensions for thinking about one's spirituality:

- Beliefs
- Spiritual practices
- Spiritual experiences

Many of these individuals would describe religion or spirituality as the most important source of strength and direction for their lives. It plays a significant and central role in the lives of many people.

(Source: "Spirituality And Trauma: Professionals Working Together," U.S. Department of Veterans Affairs (VA).)

Serious Illness May Cause Spiritual Distress

Serious illnesses like cancer may cause patients or family caregivers to have doubts about their beliefs or religious values and cause much spiritual distress. Some studies show that patients with cancer may feel that they are being punished by God or may have a loss of faith after being diagnosed. Other patients may have mild feelings of spiritual distress when coping with cancer.

Spiritual And Religious Well-Being May Help Improve Quality Of Life

It is not known for sure how spirituality and religion are related to health. Some studies show that spiritual or religious beliefs and practices create a positive mental attitude that may help a patient feel better and improve the well-being of family caregivers. Spiritual and religious well-being may help improve health and quality of life in the following ways:

- Decrease anxiety, depression, anger, and discomfort.
- Decrease the sense of isolation (feeling alone) and the risk of suicide.
- Decrease alcohol and drug abuse.
- Lower blood pressure and the risk of heart disease.
- Help the patient adjust to the effects of cancer and its treatment.
- Increase the ability to enjoy life during cancer treatment.
- Give a feeling of personal growth as a result of living with cancer.
- Increase positive feelings, including:
- Hope and optimism.
- Freedom from regret.
- Satisfaction with life.
- A sense of inner peace.
- Spiritual and religious well-being may also help a patient live longer.

Spiritual Distress May Also Affect Health

Spiritual distress may make it harder for patients to cope with cancer and cancer treatment. Healthcare providers may encourage patients to meet with experienced spiritual or religious leaders to help deal with their spiritual issues. This may improve their health, quality of life, and ability to cope.

Spiritual Assessment Might Help Doctors Understand

A spiritual assessment may include questions about the following:

- Religious denomination, if any.

- Beliefs or philosophy of life.
- Important spiritual practices or rituals.
- Using spirituality or religion as a source of strength.
- Being part of a community of support.
- Using prayer or meditation.
- Loss of faith.
- Conflicts between spiritual or religious beliefs and cancer treatments.
- Ways that healthcare providers and caregivers may help with the patient's spiritual needs.
- Concerns about death and afterlife.
- Planning for the end of life

How Healthcare Team Might Help

The healthcare team will help with a patient's spiritual needs when setting goals and planning treatment. They may help with a patient's spiritual needs in the following ways:

- Suggest goals and options for care that honor the patient's spiritual and/or religious views.
- Support the patient's use of spiritual coping during the illness.
- Encourage the patient to speak with his/her religious or spiritual leader.
- Refer the patient to a hospital chaplain or support group that can help with spiritual issues during illness.
- Refer the patient to other therapies that have been shown to increase spiritual well-being. These include mindfulness relaxation, such as yoga or meditation, or creative arts programs, such as writing, drawing, or music therapy.

Three Types Of Spirituality

We can live on junk food, at least for a while. However, junk food is not for healthy eating. Junk food is for pleasure. In time, we pay the price of our food choice. We have poorer health. In a like way, if we feed our inner spirit with pleasing but not healthy matter, over time we become poorer in spirit.

Religious Spirituality

There are three types of spirituality. There is religious spirituality. Most of us know this kind. It involves belief in a being greater than oneself, church, and prayer. Some people try to be like the masters of spirituality in their church. Other people find their spirituality in the books of religions. It does not matter where or how they find their spirituality. For many people, their religious beliefs shape and define their spiritual lives. They are inseparable.

Nonreligious Spirituality

A second type of spirituality is nonreligious spirituality. It centers on doing something positive. This gives a sense of peace in one's spirit. Nonreligious spiritual acts often mean creating things or making something by hand. This act gives a sense of satisfaction. Fans of the television show Naval Criminal Investigative Service (NCIS) may recall a scene. After Agent Gibbs solves a disturbing crime, he retreats to his basement. There he quietly, carefully works on his handmade boat. The message is simple. The act of creating something fed his soul. The acts of destruction he saw took away his sense of peace. Building something of beauty gives back his inner peace. His spirit is nourished back to health. Making the boat gives meaning and purpose to his life. This is an example of nonreligious spirituality.

Toxic Spirituality

The third kind of spirituality is toxic, or pseudo-spirituality. More often than not, this involves an action or the use of a substance. At first, this causes a good feeling, a rush. Too much use of drugs, alcohol, gambling, food, and the like all provide the person with a rush or feeling high. Even exercise, when done in excess, can make us feel good at first.

The action is repeated often to try to get back that good feeling. After all, it is only natural to seek things that make us feel good about ourselves. People want to believe that their lives have meaning. The problem comes up when such actions take over our lives. The action becomes meaning itself for us.

Medical Staff Should Respect Patient Beliefs

To help patients with spiritual needs during cancer care, medical staff will listen to the wishes of the patient.

Spirituality and religion are very personal issues. Patients should expect doctors and caregivers to respect their religious and spiritual beliefs and concerns. Patients with cancer who rely on spirituality to cope with the disease should be able to count on the healthcare team to give them support. This may include giving patients information about people or groups that can help with spiritual or religious needs. Most hospitals have chaplains, but not all outpatient settings do. Patients who do not want to discuss spirituality during cancer care should also be able to count on the healthcare team to respect their wishes.

Doctors and caregivers will try to respond to their patients' concerns, but may not take part in patients' religious practices or discuss specific religious beliefs.

> Spirituality falls under the "social" dimension of understanding health and illness. The preponderance of evidence suggests that attaining a degree of spiritual well-being may yield a positive effect on health. Whether as part of a formal religion or one's personal belief system, spiritual well-being offers one a sense of meaning, purpose, and hope. Ultimately, it may also influence the will to live.
>
> *(Source: "Sleep And Spirituality Among The Factors Being Explored In Suicide Research," U.S. Department of Veterans Affairs (VA).)*

Chapter 32

Feng Shui

Feng shui is an ancient philosophical system of Chinese origin that dates back to 1700 BCE. It is based on the concept that people who live in harmony with their environment can lead healthier, happier, more productive lives. Feng shui is the art of designing the physical environment so that it balances various elements of nature. Achieving this balance is believed to enhance the flow of *qi* (pronounced "chee"), the central energy or life force that is present in all things. When qi flows gently and smoothly through a person's surroundings, it may exert a positive influence on their health, relationships, and worldly success.

History Of Feng Shui

In ancient China, the principles of feng shui were widely used to select, orient, design, and decorate living spaces. Citizens relied upon the system to choose locations to build homes, grow crops, and bury departed family members. The dynasties that ruled over China applied this "art of placement" to the construction of palaces, government buildings, and even entire cities.

Over time, the principles associated with feng shui expanded to include nuances from astronomy, astrology, philosophy, cosmology, and metaphysics. During the Cultural Revolution of 1966–76, however, Chinese Communist leaders purged the country of many traditional elements of Chinese culture. Although the practice of feng shui was suppressed in mainland China, the discipline gained prominence in the United States and elsewhere in the world.

Principles Of Feng Shui

Wherever it is practiced, feng shui incorporates the same basic principles:

Qi. In traditional Chinese culture, qi is the life force or energy flow that permeates all living things and connects them to the natural environment. Qi is the core principle of feng shui as well as traditional Chinese medicine and martial arts. In the practice of feng shui, people strive to arrange their surroundings to remove obstructions, create harmony, and keep qi flowing smoothly.

Yin and Yang. Feng shui also incorporates the principle of polarity or duality. Under this principle, everything in nature is comprised of two opposing, yet interconnected forces. These two forces cannot exist without each other, and they can be regarded as parts of a whole circle. Yin is considered to be a female force, and it is often characterized as soft, gentle, and nurturing. Yang, on the other hand, is considered to be a male force, characterized as hard, active, and aggressive. In feng shui, people strive to balance opposing forces—light and dark, straight and curvy, etc.—in an effort to promote harmony in their environment.

Connectedness. This principle is based on the idea that the environment can influence people, just as people can influence their environment. Due to this connectedness, organizing one's surroundings through the practice of feng shui is believed to have an impact on other aspects of one's life, such as health and success.

The Five Elements. Feng shui divides the environment into five elements: fire, earth, metal, water, and wood. The five elements are believed to relate to each other as they do in nature, in what are known as productive cycles and destructive cycles. Arranging surroundings with feng shui means striving to attain balance between the various elements. When one element is emphasized too heavily, it can obstruct the flow of qi and make the surroundings feel uncomfortable. Each element is associated with a certain shape, color, and set of characteristics or attributes:

1. Fire is represented by a triangle and the color red. Among the qualities associated with the fire element are passion, enthusiasm, expressiveness, inspiration, boldness, and leadership. In the environment, objects that incorporate the fire element include candles, fireplaces, and lamps.

2. Earth is represented by a square, and its main colors are brown and yellow. It is associated with such attributes as balance, stability, grounding, and practicality. Objects that bring the earth element into the environment might include hardwood floors, granite countertops, or clay pots.

3. Metal is represented by a circle, and its main colors are silver, gold, and white. Metal energy is associated with activities of the mind, such as strength, focus, and clarity of thought. This element can be featured in the environment through the use of wrought

iron furniture or light fixtures, metal picture frames, or electronic devices like clocks or televisions.

4. Water is represented by wavy lines and the colors blue and black. It is regarded as a mystical element that symbolizes spirituality, reflection, movement, and flow. It can be incorporated into the environment in the form of water-filled glass vases, aquariums, fountains, or objects that have a swirling pattern.
5. Wood is represented by a rectangle and the color green. Among the attributes of wood energy are growth, vitality, and creativity. Objects that bring wood energy into the environment include anything made of wood, such as furniture or flooring, as well as live plants and flowers—especially bamboo.

The Bagua. The bagua is an important tool used in the practice of feng shui. It is an octagonal or rectangular chart containing nine equal spaces that correspond to the following critical aspects of life:

- Power and wealth
- Fame and reputation
- Love and relationships
- Children and legacy
- Compassion and travel
- Work and career
- Knowledge and wisdom
- Health and community
- Well-being and balance

The bagua is used to determine which physical part of a home, office, shop, or restaurant relates to each attribute. This information can help people decide how to decorate or place favorite personal possessions within a space in order to enhance the flow of qi.

The first step in using the bagua involves orienting it to the space, with the main entrance in the middle of the bottom row. Next, feng shui experts suggest conceptualizing the floor plan of the space as nine squares that match the ones on the bagua. Finally, they recommend decorating and accessorizing each area with objects that activate the specific energy or attributes of the corresponding square on the bagua. For example, diplomas and trophies should be placed in the area that represents fame and reputation, while family photos and children's drawings should be placed in the area that represents children and legacy. Proponents of feng shui believe that people who use these principles to organize their surroundings will achieve greater balance and experience positive changes in their lives.

References

1. Jones, Katina Z. *The Everything Feng Shui Book,* New York: F+W Media, 2011.
2. Olmstead, Carol. "Basics," Feng Shui for Real Life, 2015.

Chapter 33

Shiatsu

Shiatsu, which is a Japanese word meaning "finger pressure," is a form of therapeutic bodywork. Practitioners use their fingers, thumbs, and palms to knead, press, tap, and stretch various parts of the body in a rhythmic sequence. In most forms of shiatsu, the goal is to correct imbalances in the flow of energy through the body, known as *qi* (pronounced "chee") in Japanese and Chinese medical traditions. According to these traditions, obstructions or deficiencies in the qi can contribute to many chronic health issues, such as headaches, muscular pain, digestive problems, or frequent colds. Shiatsu therapists use manual techniques to access the qi, harmonize the flow of energy through the body, and thus restore the client to good health.

History Of Shiatsu

The person often credited as the founder of modern shiatsu therapy is Tokujiro Namikoshi, who was born in Japan in 1905. He began using hands-on therapy techniques at the age of seven to treat his mother's rheumatoid arthritis. He eventually developed a theory of bodywork that he called shiatsu and established a school to train shiatsu therapists. Namikoshi introduced shiatsu to the United States in the 1950s, and from there it spread around the world. Although shiatsu evolved from anma, a massage system popularized in the 1600s by acupuncturist Sugiyama Waichi, it integrated this traditional Japanese form of manual therapy with modern medical knowledge. The Japanese Ministry of Health recognized shiatsu as a distinct form of therapeutic treatment in 1964.

Over the years, many shiatsu practitioners developed their own therapeutic styles. Some approaches emphasize stimulation of acupressure points, while others concentrate on influencing the flow of qi. Although the techniques may differ slightly, they all share the same basic goals. Some of the common variations include:

- Five Element Shiatsu
- Hara Shiatsu
- Macrobiotic Shiatsu
- Meridian Shiatsu
- Oha Shiatsu
- Quantum Shiatsu
- Tao Shiatsu
- Tsubo Shiatsu
- Water Shiatsu
- Zen Shiatsu

The Shiatsu Treatment Process

Regardless of the style used, a shiatsu treatment typically begins with an assessment of state of the client's qi. The practitioner performs this evaluation in order to determine what obstructions or sources of imbalance might be present. This process allows the therapist to design a treatment plan that will address the problems, restore the balance, and improve the client's health.

Following the initial assessment, the practitioner uses manual techniques—including pressing, kneading, rubbing, tapping, and stretching—to access the client's qi. The qi is believed to flow through pathways in the body called meridians. Practitioners attempt to influence the flow of energy by manipulating locations known as vital points. If the client is experiencing a great deal of stress or anxiety, the therapist may employ techniques designed to disperse energy. On the other hand, if the client is experiencing fatigue or depression, the practitioner may use techniques designed to restore energy.

Unlike some other types of massage therapy, shiatsu is performed through clothing and without the use of oils. The person undergoing treatment usually lies on a low massage table or on a pad on the floor. A typical session lasts between 60 and 90 minutes. Although shiatsu is considered a low-risk treatment, it may not be appropriate for people who have recently undergone surgery, have skin rashes, open wounds, or injuries, or who are in the advanced stages of pregnancy.

Research On Shiatsu

Most people find shiatsu therapy to be very soothing and relaxing. Anecdotal evidence suggests that it can offer some health benefits, such as alleviating pain from injuries or arthritis and reducing the psychological stress associated with illness. Proponents claim that it is also effective in relieving headaches, reducing anxiety, enhancing sleep, improving digestion, and treating the symptoms of premenstrual syndrome.

While shiatsu may aid in the healing process for some patients, doctors emphasize that it should complement, rather than replace, appropriate medical treatment. The mainstream medical community generally rejects the idea that shiatsu can effectively prevent, diagnose, or treat potentially serious medical conditions. Critics argue that there is no scientific evidence to support the existence of qi or the claim that shiatsu can improve the function of bodily systems.

References

1. Canadian Shiatsu Society of British Columbia. "About Shiatsu," n.d.
2. Pelava, Cari Johnson. "What Is Shiatsu?" *Taking Charge of Your Health and Well-Being,* Center for Spirituality and Healing, University of Minnesota, 2013.

Chapter 34

Tai Chi And Qi Gong

What Are Tai Chi And Qi Gong?

Tai chi and qi gong are centuries old, related mind and body practices. They involve certain postures and gentle movements with mental focus, breathing, and relaxation. The movements can be adapted or practiced while walking, standing, or sitting. In contrast to qi gong, tai chi movements, if practiced quickly, can be a form of combat or self-defense.

Tai chi is sometimes referred to as "moving meditation." There are many types of tai chi. They typically combine slow movements with breathing patterns and mental focus and relaxation. Movements may be done while walking, standing, or sitting. While more research is needed, studies suggest that it may have many health benefits. Research suggests that practicing tai chi might help improve posture and confidence, how you think and manage emotions, and your quality of life. Studies have found that it may help people with fibromyalgia sleep better and cope with pain, fatigue, and depression. Regular practice may also improve quality of life and mood in people with chronic heart failure or cancer.

(Source: "Tai Chi And Your Health—A Modern Take On An Ancient Practice," NIH News in Health, *National Institutes of Health (NIH).)*

What The Science Says About The Effectiveness Of Tai Chi And Qi Gong

Research findings suggest that practicing tai chi may improve balance and stability in older people and those with Parkinson, reduce pain from knee osteoarthritis, help people cope with

About This Chapter: This chapter includes text excerpted from "Tai Chi and Qi Gong: In Depth," National Center for Complementary and Integrative Health (NCCIH), October 2016.

fibromyalgia and back pain, and promote quality of life and mood in people with heart failure and cancer. There's been less research on the effects of qi gong, but some studies suggest it may reduce chronic neck pain (although results are mixed) and pain from fibromyalgia. Qi gong also may help to improve general quality of life.

Both also may offer psychological benefits, such as reducing anxiety. However, differences in how the research on anxiety was conducted make it difficult to draw firm conclusions about this.

Falling And Balance

Exercise programs, including tai chi, may reduce falling and the fear of falling in people. Tai chi also may be more effective than other forms of exercise for improving balance and stability in people with Parkinson disease.

- A review determined that tai chi, as well as other group and home-based activity programs (which often include balance and strength training exercises) effectively reduced falling in people, and tai chi significantly reduced the risk of falling. But the reviewers also found that tai chi was less effective in older people who were at higher risk of falling.
- Fear of falling can have a serious impact on a person's health and life. In a review, researchers suggested that various types of exercise, including tai chi, may reduce the fear of falling among people.
- Findings from a clinical trial with 195 people showed that practicing tai chi improved balance and stability better than resistance training or stretching in people with mild to moderate Parkinson disease. A follow-up analysis showed that people who practiced tai chi were more likely to continue exercising during the 3 months following the study compared with those who participated in resistance training or stretching.

For Pain (Knee Osteoarthritis, Fibromyalgia, Chronic Neck Pain)

There's some evidence that practicing tai chi may help people manage pain associated with knee osteoarthritis (a breakdown of cartilage in the knee that allows leg bones to rub together), fibromyalgia (a disorder that causes muscle pain and fatigue), and back pain. Qi gong may offer some benefit for chronic neck pain, but results are mixed.

Knee Osteoarthritis

- Results of a small, the National Center for Complementary and Integrative Health (NCCIH) funded clinical trial involving 40 participants with knee osteoarthritis suggested that practicing tai chi reduced pain and improved function better than an education and stretching program.
- An analysis of seven small and moderately sized clinical studies concluded that a 12-week course of tai chi reduced pain and improved function in people with this condition.

Fibromyalgia

- Results from a small NCCIH supported clinical trial suggested that practicing tai chi was more effective than wellness education and stretching in helping people with fibromyalgia sleep better and cope with pain, fatigue, and depression. After 12 weeks, those who practiced tai chi also had better scores on a survey designed to measure a person's ability to carry out certain daily activities such as walking, housecleaning, shopping, and preparing a meal. The benefits of tai chi also appeared to last longer.
- A small NCCIH supported trial suggested that combining tai chi movements with mindfulness allowed people with fibromyalgia to work through the discomfort they may feel during exercise, allowing them to take advantage of the benefits of physical activity.
- Results of a randomized clinical trial with 100 participants suggested that practicing qi gong reduced pain and improved sleep, the ability to do daily activities, and mental function. The researchers also observed that most improvements were still apparent after 6 months.

Chronic Neck Pain

- Research results on the effectiveness of qi gong for chronic neck pain are mixed, but the people who were studied and the way the studies were done were quite different.
- A clinical study by German researchers showed no benefit of qi gong or exercise compared with no therapy in 117 elderly adults (mostly women) with, on average, a 20-year history of chronic neck pain. Study participants had 24 exercise or qi gong sessions over 3 months.

- In another study, some of the same researchers observed that qi gong was just as effective as exercise therapy (and both were more effective than no therapy) in relieving neck pain in the 123 middle aged adults (mostly women) who had chronic neck pain for an average of 3 years. Exercise therapy included throwing and catching a ball, rowing and climbing movements, arm swinging, and stretching, among other activities. People in the study had 18 exercise or qi gong sessions over 6 months.

For Mental Health And Cognitive Function

- While a range of research has suggested that exercise helps reduce depression and anxiety, the role of tai chi and qi gong for these and other mental health problems is less clear. However, there is evidence that tai chi may boost brain function and reasoning ability in older people.
- NCCIH supported research suggested that practicing tai chi may help reduce stress, anxiety, and depression, and also improve mood and self-esteem. However, in their other review, which included 40 studies with more than 3,800 participants, the researchers noted that they couldn't develop firm conclusions because of differences in study designs.
- In a NCCIH supported review, researchers found that the results from 29 studies with more than 2,500 participants didn't offer clear evidence about the effectiveness of tai chi and qi gong on such psychological factors as anxiety, depression, stress, mood, and self-esteem. But the researchers noted that most of these studies weren't looking primarily at psychological distress and didn't intentionally recruit participants with mental health issues.
- Results from another NCCIH supported review suggested that practicing tai chi may enhance the ability to reason, plan, remember, and solve problems in older people without evidence of significant cognitive impairment. The data also indicated that tai chi boosted cognitive ability in people who showed signs of mild cognitive impairment to dementia, but to a lesser degree than in those with no signs of cognitive impairment.

For Quality Of Life

Much research suggests that physical activity enhances quality of life. Health providers who treat people with cancer often recommend exercise to reduce illness related fatigue and improve quality of life. Some studies also suggest that physical activity helps people with heart disease and other chronic illnesses.

Cancer

- Research results indicated that practicing qi gong may improve quality of life, mood, fatigue, and inflammation in adults with different types of cancer, compared with those receiving usual care. However, the researchers suggested that the attention received by the qi gong participants may have contributed to the positive study findings.

Heart Disease

Regular practice of tai chi may improve quality of life and mood in people with chronic heart failure, according to a clinical trial funded by NCCIH.

Results from a small study suggested that practicing tai chi improved the ability to exercise and may be an option as cardiac rehabilitation for people who have had a heart attack.

Other

A NCCIH supported research review examined the effects of tai chi and qi gong on the quality of life of adults who were healthy, elderly, were breast cancer or stroke survivors, or had a chronic disease. The analysis suggested that practicing tai chi or qi gong may improve quality of life in healthy and chronically ill people.

What The Science Says About Safety Of Tai Chi And Qi Gong

Tai chi and qi gong appear to be safe practices. One NCCIH supported review noted that tai chi is unlikely to result in serious injury but it may be associated with minor aches and pains. Women who are pregnant should talk with their healthcare providers before beginning tai chi, qi gong, or any other exercise program.

Is Tai Chi Right For Me?

- Talk with your healthcare provider about your physical activity and limits. Ask whether tai chi might be a good option for you.
- Look for classes based on your age and health. Some classes may be geared toward college students and stress management; others may be designed for folks over age 60 with particular medical conditions.
- Observe several teachers and classes to find a fit for you. There are different teaching styles, levels, and ways to practice tai chi.

- Don't be discouraged if you can't do all the movements. Think about the potential health benefits, and try to be patient with yourself.

Everyone has to start somewhere!

(Source: "Tai Chi And Your Health—A Modern Take On An Ancient Practice," NIH News in Health, *National Institutes of Health (NIH).)*

Training, Licensing, And Certification

Tai chi instructors don't have to be licensed, and the practice isn't regulated by the Federal Government or individual states. There's no national standard for qi gong certification. Various tai chi and qi gong organizations offer training and certification programs—with differing criteria and levels of certification for instructors.

Chapter 35

Tui Na

Tui na is a form of massage therapy that originated in China around 2,500 years ago. Its name comes from the Chinese words for two of the motions commonly used by practitioners, *tui* (meaning "push") and *na* ("squeeze"). Tui na incorporates elements from several different forms of traditional Chinese medicine and martial arts, including qi gong, shiatsu, acupuncture, fire cupping, and tai chi.

Although it employs manual manipulation techniques similar to those used in other types of body massage—such as pressing, kneading, tapping, rolling, gliding, and shaking—tui na tends to focus on identifying and addressing specific problems rather than on promoting simple relaxation. The goal for the tui na therapist is to find and correct imbalances in the flow of energy through the patient's body, known as *qi* (pronounced "chee"). According to traditional Chinese medicine, obstructions or deficiencies in the qi can contribute to many chronic health issues. Tui na therapists use manual techniques to access the qi, harmonize the flow of energy through the body, and thus restore the patient to good health.

The Tui Na Treatment Process

Proponents of tui na believe that the qi must be in balance for a person to have positive energy and enjoy good health. The tui na treatment process thus focuses on enhancing the flow of qi through the body in channels called meridians. Therapists are trained to access the qi by massaging vital points along the meridians. They may employ a variety of manual techniques designed to remove obstructions in the flow of energy, such as kneading, rolling, rubbing, gliding, pulling, rocking, rotating, vibrating, and shaking. Some tui na practitioners also incorporate acupressure or spinal manipulation techniques into the treatment process.

A typical tui na therapy session lasts between 30 and 60 minutes. The client usually wears loose clothing and lies on a massage table or floor mat. The practitioner begins by examining the client to identify problem areas, whether specific pain sites or obstructions in the flow of qi. Then the therapist applies manual massage techniques to acupressure points, energy meridians, and muscles and joints to treat the problems. The client usually feels relaxed but energized at the end of the treatment. Depending on the severity of the problems, the client may need to return for additional sessions.

Benefits Of Tui Na

Proponents claim that tui na massage therapy can lead to improvements in many different health conditions, including arthritis, sciatica, muscle spasms, chronic pain, insomnia, digestive problems, constipation, headaches, and stress. They believe that restoring the free flow of energy through the body relaxes muscles, relieves pain, improves circulation, and creates a feeling of vitality and emotional well-being.

While tui na may aid in the healing process for some patients, doctors warn that it should only complement, rather than replace, conventional medical treatment for potentially serious health conditions. Critics argue that there is no scientific evidence to support the existence of qi or the claim that tui na can improve the function of bodily systems. In addition, since tui na is more vigorous and intense than many other forms of massage, it may not be appropriate for everyone.

References

1. Hafner, Christopher. "Tui Na," Center for Spirituality and Healing, University of Minnesota, 2013.
2. Henderson, Jan. "What Is Tui Na?" Balance Flow Health and Bodyworks, 2014.
3. Pacific College of Oriental Medicine. "Benefits of Tui Na Massage," 2014.

Chapter 36

Yoga

Yoga is a mind and body practice with historical origins in ancient Indian philosophy. Like other meditative movement practices used for health purposes, various styles of yoga typically combine physical postures, breathing techniques, and meditation or relaxation.

Yoga in its full form combines physical postures, breathing exercises, meditation, and a distinct philosophy. There are numerous styles of yoga. Hatha yoga, commonly practiced in the United States and Europe, emphasizes postures, breathing exercises, and meditation. Hatha yoga styles include Ananda, Anusara, Ashtanga, Bikram, Iyengar, Kripalu, Kundalini, Viniyoga, and others.

Fun Facts

- The word yoga comes from an ancient language and means yoke or unite—to bring together your body, mind, and spirit.
- A "yogin" is a male student while a "yogini" is a female student.
- Many yoga poses are based on animals and the different postures they do in nature.
- More than 6 million people practice yoga including Madonna, Kareem Abdul Jabar, and Michelle Pfeiffer.

(Source: "BAM, Physical Activity, Yoga," Centers for Disease Control and Prevention (CDC).)

About This Chapter: This chapter includes text excerpted from "Yoga: In Depth," National Center for Complementary and Integrative Health (NCCIH), June 2013. Reviewed January 2018.

Side Effects And Risks

- Yoga is generally low impact and safe for healthy people when practiced appropriately under the guidance of a well-trained instructor.
- Overall, those who practice yoga have a low rate of side effects, and the risk of serious injury from yoga is quite low. However, certain types of stroke as well as pain from nerve damage are among the rare possible side effects of practicing yoga.
- Women who are pregnant and people with certain medical conditions, such as high blood pressure, glaucoma (a condition in which fluid pressure within the eye slowly increases and may damage the eye's optic nerve), and sciatica (pain, weakness, numbing, or tingling that may extend from the lower back to the calf, foot, or even the toes), should modify or avoid some yoga poses.

Use Of Yoga For Health In The United States

According to the 2007 National Health Interview Survey (NHIS), which included a comprehensive survey on the use of complementary health approaches (CHA) by Americans, yoga is the sixth most commonly used complementary health practice among adults. More than 13 million adults practiced yoga in the previous year, and between the 2002 and 2007 NHIS, use of yoga among adults increased by 1 percent (or approximately 3 million people). The 2007 survey also found that more than 1.5 million children practiced yoga in the previous year.

Many people who practice yoga do so to maintain their health and well-being, improve physical fitness, relieve stress, and enhance quality of life. In addition, they may be addressing specific health conditions, such as back pain, neck pain, arthritis, and anxiety.

What The Science Says About Yoga

Research suggests that a carefully adapted set of yoga poses may reduce low back pain and improve function. Other studies also suggest that practicing yoga (as well as other forms of regular exercise) might improve quality of life; reduce stress; lower heart rate; and blood pressure; help relieve anxiety, depression, and insomnia; and improve overall physical fitness, strength, and flexibility. But some research suggests yoga may not improve asthma, and studies looking at yoga and arthritis have had mixed results.

- One National Center for Complementary and Integrative Health (NCCIH) funded study of 90 people with chronic low back pain found that participants who practiced Iyengar yoga had significantly less disability, pain, and depression after 6 months.

- In a study, also funded by NCCIH, researchers compared yoga with conventional stretching exercises or a self-care book in 228 adults with chronic low back pain. The results showed that both yoga and stretching were more effective than a self-care book for improving function and reducing symptoms due to chronic low back pain.
- Conclusions from another study of 313 adults with chronic or recurring low back pain suggested that 12 weekly yoga classes resulted in better function than usual medical care.

National Institutes of Health (NIH)-funded researchers have been looking for new ways to treat long-lasting low-back pain. A new study shows that yoga may help relieve moderate to severe low-back pain. The research team recruited 320 people with chronic low-back pain from diverse backgrounds and underserved communities. The results suggested that a structured yoga class may be an option for treating chronic low-back pain. All three groups reported improvement in physical function and pain reduction.

(Source: "Yoga May Help Treat Back Pain," NIH News in Health, *National Institutes of Health (NIH).)*

However, studies show that certain health conditions may not benefit from yoga.

- A systematic review of clinical studies suggests that there is no sound evidence that yoga improves asthma.
- A review of the literature reports that few published studies have looked at yoga and arthritis, and of those that have, results are inconclusive. The two main types of arthritis—osteoarthritis and rheumatoid arthritis—are different conditions, and the effects of yoga may not be the same for each. In addition, the reviewers suggested that even if a study showed that yoga helped osteoarthritic finger joints, it may not help osteoarthritic knee joints.

Training, Licensing, And Certification

There are many training programs for yoga teachers throughout the country. These programs range from a few days to more than 2 years. Standards for teacher training and certification differ depending on the style of yoga.

There are organizations that register yoga teachers and training programs that have complied with a certain curriculum and educational standards. For example, one nonprofit group (the Yoga Alliance) requires at least 200 hours of training, with a specified number of hours in areas including techniques, teaching methodology, anatomy, physiology, and philosophy.

Most yoga therapist training programs involve 500 hours or more. The training standards of the International Association of Yoga Therapists (IAYT) are competency based and require at least 800 hours after a basic 200 hours teacher training program.

If You Are Considering Practicing Yoga

- Do not use yoga to replace conventional medical care or to postpone seeing a healthcare provider about pain or any other medical condition.
- If you have a medical condition, talk to your healthcare provider before starting yoga.
- Ask a trusted source (such as your healthcare provider or a nearby hospital) to recommend a yoga practitioner. Find out about the training and experience of any practitioner you are considering.
- Everyone's body is different, and yoga postures should be modified based on individual abilities. Carefully selecting an instructor who is experienced with and attentive to your needs is an important step toward helping you practice yoga safely. Ask about the physical demands of the type of yoga in which you are interested and inform your yoga instructor about any medical issues you have.
- Carefully think about the type of yoga you are interested in. For example, hot yoga (such as Bikram yoga) may involve standing and moving in humid environments with temperatures as high as 105°F. Because such settings may be physically stressful, people who practice hot yoga should take certain precautions. These include drinking water before, during, and after a hot yoga practice and wearing suitable clothing. People with conditions that may be affected by excessive heat, such as heart disease, lung disease, and a prior history of heatstroke may want to avoid this form of yoga. Women who are pregnant may want to check with their healthcare providers before starting hot yoga.
- Tell all your healthcare providers about any complementary health approaches you use. Give them a full picture of what you do to manage your health. This will help ensure coordinated and safe care.

Part Five

Biologically Based Practices

Chapter 37

Nutrition And Health

Importance Of Good Nutrition

Your food choices each day affect your health—how you feel today, tomorrow, and in the future.

Good nutrition is an important part of leading a healthy life style. Combined with physical activity, your diet can help you to reach and maintain a healthy weight, reduce your risk of chronic diseases (like heart disease and cancer), and promote your overall health.

Nutrition

Food provides the energy and nutrients you need to be healthy. Nutrients include proteins, carbohydrates, fats, vitamins, minerals, and water.

Healthy eating is not hard. The key is to:

- Eat a variety of foods, including vegetables, fruits, and whole-grain products
- Eat lean meats, poultry, fish, beans, and low-fat dairy products
- Drink lots of water
- Limit salt, sugar, alcohol, saturated fat, and *trans* fat in your diet

(Source: "Nutrition," MedlinePlus, National Institutes of Health (NIH).)

About This Chapter: Text beginning with the heading "Importance Of Good Nutrition" is excerpted from "Importance Of Good Nutrition," U.S. Department of Health and Human Services (HHS), January 26, 2017; Text beginning with the heading "Eat The Right Amount Of Calories For You" is excerpted from "Dietary Guidelines For Americans—Let's Eat For The Health Of It," U.S. Department of Agriculture (USDA), June 2011. Reviewed January 2018.

The Impact Of Nutrition On Your Health

Unhealthy eating habits have contributed to the obesity epidemic in the United States: approximately 17 percent (or 12.5 million) of children and adolescents aged 2–19 years are obese. Even for people at a healthy weight, a poor diet is associated with major health risks that can cause illness and even death. These include heart disease, hypertension (high blood pressure), type 2 diabetes, osteoporosis, and certain types of cancer. By making smart food choices, you can help protect yourself from these health problems.

The risk factors for adult chronic diseases, like hypertension and type 2 diabetes, are increasingly seen in younger ages, often a result of unhealthy eating habits and increased weight gain. Dietary habits established in childhood often carry into adulthood, so teaching children how to eat healthy at a young age will help them stay healthy throughout their life.

The link between good nutrition and healthy weight, reduced chronic disease risk, and overall health is too important to ignore. By taking steps to eat healthy, you'll be on your way to getting the nutrients your body needs to stay healthy, active, and strong. As with physical activity, making small changes in your diet can go a long way, and it's easier than you think!

How To Eat Healthy

It's easier than you think to start eating healthy! Take small steps each week to improve your nutrition and move toward a healthier you.

Eat The Right Amount Of Calories For You

Everyone has a personal calorie limit. Staying within yours can help you get to or maintain a healthy weight. People who are successful at managing their weight have found ways to keep track of how much they eat in a day, even if they don't count every calorie.

Enjoy your food, but eat less.

- Get your personal daily calorie limit at www.ChooseMyPlate.gov and keep that number in mind when deciding what to eat.
- Think before you eat—is it worth the calories?
- Avoid oversized portions.
- Use a smaller plate, bowl, and glass.
- Stop eating when you are satisfied, not full.

Cook more often at home, where you are in control of what's in your food. When eating out, choose lower calorie menu options.

- Check posted calorie amounts.
- Choose dishes that include vegetables, fruits, and/or whole grains.
- Order a smaller portion or share when eating out.

Write down what you eat to keep track of how much you eat. If you drink alcoholic beverages, do so sensibly—limit to 1 drink a day for women or to 2 drinks a day for men.

The Caloric Balance Equation

Whether you need to lose weight, maintain your ideal weight, or gain weight, the main message is—calories count! Weight management is all about balancing the number of calories you take in with the number your body uses or "burns off."

- A calorie is a unit of energy supplied by food and beverages. A calorie is a calorie regardless of its source. Carbohydrates, fats, sugars, and proteins all contain calories.
- If your body does not use calories, they are stored as fat.
- Caloric balance is like a scale. To remain in balance and maintain your body weight, the calories consumed must be balanced by the calories used in normal body functions, daily activities, and exercise.

(Source: "Healthy Weight—Finding A Balance," Centers for Disease Control and Prevention (CDC).)

Use Food Labels To Help You Make Better Choices

Most packaged foods have a Nutrition Facts label and an ingredients list. For a healthier you, use this tool to make smart food choices quickly and easily.

Check for calories. Be sure to look at the serving size and how many servings you are actually consuming. If you double the servings you eat, you double the calories.

Choose foods with lower calories, saturated fat, *trans* fat, and sodium. Check for added sugars using the ingredients list. When a sugar is close to first on the ingredients list, the food is high in added sugars. Some names for added sugars include sucrose, glucose, high fructose corn syrup, corn syrup, maple syrup, and fructose

> You can enjoy your meals while making small shifts to the amounts and types of food on your plate. Healthy meals start with a variety and balance of foods from each food group. Aim to consume less sodium, saturated fat, and added sugars
>
> *(Source: "Enjoy Your Food, But Eat Less," ChooseMyPlate.gov, U.S. Department of Agriculture (USDA).)*

Be Physically Active Your Way

Pick activities that you like and start by doing what you can, at least 10 minutes at a time. Every bit adds up, and the health benefits increase as you spend more time being active.

Chapter 38

Clinical Nutrition

Nutrition And Health Are Closely Related

Over the past century, essential nutrient deficiencies have dramatically decreased, many infectious diseases have been conquered, and the majority of the U.S. population can now anticipate a long and productive life. However, as infectious disease rates have dropped, the rates of noncommunicable diseases—specifically, chronic diet-related diseases—have risen, due in part to changes in lifestyle behaviors. A history of poor eating and physical activity patterns have a cumulative effect and have contributed to significant nutrition- and physical activity-related health challenges that now face the U.S. population. About half of all American adults—117 million individuals—have one or more preventable chronic diseases, many of which are related to poor quality eating patterns and physical inactivity. These include cardiovascular disease, high blood pressure, type 2 diabetes, some cancers, and poor bone health. More than two-thirds of adults and nearly one-third of children and youth are overweight or

---

About This Chapter: Text under the heading "Nutrition And Health Are Closely Related" is excerpted from "Introduction: Nutrition And Health Are Closely Related," Office of Disease Prevention and Health Promotion (ODPHP), U.S. Department of Health and Human Services (HHS), December 15, 2015; Text under the heading "Nutrition And Public Health" is excerpted from "Nutrition And Public Health," U.S. Department of Agriculture (USDA), October 5, 2017; Text under the heading "Role Of Clinical Nutrition In Healthcare" is excerpted from "How Your Eating Habits Affect Your Health," *NIH News in Health*, National Institutes of Health (NIH), May 2017; Text under the heading "What Are Nutritional Supplements?" is excerpted from "FDA 101: Dietary Supplements," U.S. Food and Drug Administration (FDA), July 15, 2015; Text under the heading "How Do Vitamins And Minerals Work?" is excerpted from "Healthy Eating—Vitamins And Minerals," National Institute on Aging (NIA), National Institutes of Health (NIH), June 17, 2017; Text under the heading "Who Is A Registered Dietitian Nutritionist?" is excerpted from "How To Contact A VA Dietitian Nutritionist," U.S. Department of Veterans Affairs (VA), September 2, 2015; Text under the heading "Nutrition Care Process" is excerpted from "Nutrition Department—Clinical Nutrition Services," Clinical Center, National Institutes of Health (NIH), July 19, 2017.

obese. These high rates of overweight and obesity and chronic disease have persisted for more than two decades and come not only with increased health risks, but also at high cost. In 2008, the medical costs associated with obesity were estimated to be $147 billion. In 2012, the total estimated cost of diagnosed diabetes was $245 billion, including $176 billion in direct medical costs and $69 billion in decreased productivity.

Nutrition And Public Health

Public health providers across the spectrum, from individual physicians to community clinics and hospitals, are realizing that treating food insecurity and poor nutrition as a health issue can lead to better health outcomes for patients, improvements in community health, and cost savings. Increasingly, nonprofit hospitals are engaging in proactive work to address food insecurity and nutrition, not only among their own patients, but more broadly as a part of their "community benefit" programs to promote population health in the communities where they are located. These programs are leveraging and increasing the impact of the U.S. Department of Agriculture (USDA) Food and Nutrition Service (FNS). They use our nation's core nutrition programs to address food insecurity and improve nutrition.

New Models Are Emerging That View Hunger As A Health Issue

There are clear associations between food insecurity and poor health status, just like there are between food insecurity and lower scores on physical and mental health exams. Those living in food insecure households consume fewer servings of fruits, vegetables, and whole grains, and more sugar, fat, and salt. These dietary shortfalls are linked to chronic diseases, including diabetes, cardiovascular disease, and cancer. Given their vulnerability, the elderly and children suffer the greatest impact.

Role Of Clinical Nutrition In Healthcare

A new study shows how the things you eat can influence your risk of dying from heart disease, stroke, or type 2 diabetes. The findings suggest ways to change your eating habits to improve your health. Experts already know that a healthy eating plan includes vegetables, fruits, whole grains, and fat-free or low-fat dairy products. A healthy diet also includes lean meats, poultry, fish, beans, eggs, and nuts. It limits saturated and *trans* fats, sodium, and added sugars.

National Institutes of Health (NIH)-funded scientists analyzed how these 10 dietary factors affect your risk of death from heart disease, stroke, and type 2 diabetes. These are known as cardiometabolic diseases. The team relied on data from the Centers for Disease Control and Prevention's (CDC) National Health and Nutrition Examination Survey (NHANES) and national mortality data.

The scientists found that risk of death from the 3 diseases was higher for those who consumed too much sodium, processed meat, sugar-sweetened beverages, and unprocessed red meat. Risk of death was also higher among those who didn't eat enough nuts and seeds, seafood omega-3 fats, vegetables, fruits, whole grains, or polyunsaturated fats. According to the analysis, nearly half (45%) of deaths in 2012 from the 3 diseases was associated with too much or too little of these 10 dietary factors.

"This study establishes the number of cardiometabolic deaths that can be linked to Americans' eating habits, and the number is large," explains Dr. David Goff, a heart disease and public health expert at NIH. "Second, it shows how recent reductions in those deaths relate to improvements in diet, and this relationship is strong. There is much work to be done in preventing heart disease, but we also know that better dietary habits can improve our health quickly, and we can act on that knowledge by making and building on small changes that add up over time."

What Are Nutritional Supplements?

The law defines dietary supplements in part as products taken by mouth that contain a "dietary ingredient." Dietary ingredients include vitamins, minerals, amino acids, and herbs or botanicals, as well as other substances that can be used to supplement the diet.

Dietary supplements come in many forms, including tablets, capsules, powders, energy bars, and liquids. These products are available in stores throughout the United States, as well as on the Internet. They are labeled as dietary supplements and include among others

- vitamin and mineral products.
- "botanical" or herbal products—These come in many forms and may include plant materials, algae, macroscopic fungi, or a combination of these materials.
- amino acid products—Amino acids are known as the building blocks of proteins and play a role in metabolism.
- enzyme supplements—Enzymes are complex proteins that speed up biochemical reactions.

People use dietary supplements for a wide assortment of reasons. Some seek to compensate for diets, medical conditions, or eating habits that limit the intake of essential vitamins and nutrients. Other people look to them to boost energy or to get a good night's sleep. Postmenopausal women consider using them to counter a sudden drop in estrogen levels.

How Do Vitamins And Minerals Work?

Vitamins help your body grow and work the way it should. There are 13 vitamins—vitamins C, A, D, E, K, and the B vitamins (thiamine, riboflavin, niacin, pantothenic acid, biotin, B6, B12, and folate). Vitamins have different jobs—helping you resist infections, keeping your nerves healthy, and helping your body get energy from food or your blood to clot properly. It is usually better to get the nutrients you need from food, rather than a pill. That's because nutrient-dense foods contain other things that are good for you, like fiber. Look for foods fortified with certain vitamins and minerals, like some B vitamins, calcium, and vitamin D. That means those nutrients are added to the foods to help you meet your needs. Minerals also help your body function. Some minerals, like iodine and fluoride, are only needed in very small quantities. Others, such as calcium, magnesium, and potassium, are needed in larger amounts. As with vitamins, if you eat a varied diet, you will probably get enough of most minerals.

Who Is A Registered Dietitian Nutritionist?

A Registered dietitian nutritionist (RDN) is a trained nutritional professional who has met the minimum academic and professional requirements to qualify for the credential "RDN." Dietitian nutritionist encourage everyone to adopt eating and physical activity plans that are focused on consuming fewer calories, making informed food choices, getting daily exercise in order to achieve and maintain a healthy weight, and to reduce the risk of chronic disease and promote overall health.

Some of the areas a dietitian nutritionist can help you in managing your health:

- Diabetes
- Gastrointestinal problems
- Heart disease
- Kidney disease
- Managing the side effects of cancer
- Weight management

Nutrition Care Process

Nutrition Assessment

For patients determined to be at nutrition risk, dietitians use innovative assessment and evaluation techniques to customize the nutrition care process for each individual. Dietitians gather information from the following areas to complete the nutrition assessment:

- Food/nutrition–related history
- Biochemical data, medical tests, and procedures
- Anthropometric measurements
- Nutrition-focused physical findings
- Client history

Nutrition Diagnosis

Dietitians use the information obtained during the nutrition assessment to identify and label a specific nutrition diagnosis (problem) by using standardized language. These problems are usually categorized into one or more of three areas: Intake, Clinical, and Behavioral-Environmental.

Nutrition Intervention

Dietitians develop specific actions to remedy a nutrition diagnosis/problem. Working with patients and the healthcare team, dietitians establish mutually agreed upon interventions and goals. These interventions include: nutrition education, nutrition counseling, coordination of care and provision of specific recommendations regarding food and/or nutrients. Dietitians skilled in nutrition support can provide guidance and recommendations for enteral and parenteral feeding.

Nutrition Monitoring And Evaluation

Dietitians monitor and quantify the progress made by patients in meeting their nutrition care goals and determine whether the nutrition intervention is successful. Dietitians monitor outcomes by selecting appropriate indicators and revise the interventions and goals as needed based on patient progress.

Chapter 39

Dietary Supplements

Dietary supplements can be beneficial to your health—but taking supplements can also involve health risks. The U.S. Food and Drug Administration (FDA) does not have the authority to review dietary supplement products for safety and effectiveness before they are marketed.

You've heard about them, may have used them, and may have even recommended them to friends or family. While some dietary supplements are well understood and established, others need further study.

Before making decisions about whether to take a supplement, talk to your healthcare provider. They can help you achieve a balance between the foods and nutrients you personally need.

What Are Dietary Supplements?

Dietary supplements include such ingredients as vitamins, minerals, herbs, amino acids, and enzymes. Dietary supplements are marketed in forms such as tablets, capsules, softgels, gelcaps, powders, and liquids.

About This Chapter: Text in this chapter begins with excerpts from "Dietary Supplements: What You Need To Know," U.S. Food and Drug Administration (FDA), November 29, 2017; Text beginning with the heading "Making Informed Decisions And Evaluating Information" is excerpted from "Tips For Dietary Supplement Users," U.S. Food and Drug Administration (FDA), November 29, 2017.

Are Dietary Supplements Different From Foods And Drugs?

Although dietary supplements are regulated by the FDA as foods, they are regulated differently from other foods and from drugs. Whether a product is classified as a dietary supplement, conventional food, or drug is based on its intended use. Most often, classification as a dietary supplement is determined by the information that the manufacturer provides on the product label or in accompanying literature, although many food and dietary supplement product labels do not include this information.

(Source: "Dietary Supplements—Background Information," Office of Dietary Supplements (ODS), National Institutes of Health (NIH).)

What Are The Benefits Of Dietary Supplements?

Some supplements can help assure that you get enough of the vital substances the body needs to function; others may help reduce the risk of disease. But supplements should not replace complete meals which are necessary for a healthful diet—so, be sure you eat a variety of foods as well.

Unlike drugs, supplements are not permitted to be marketed for the purpose of treating, diagnosing, preventing, or curing diseases. That means supplements should not make disease claims, such as "lowers high cholesterol" or "treats heart disease." Claims like these cannot be legitimately made for dietary supplements.

Nearly 12 percent of children (about one in nine) in the United States use a complementary health approach, such as dietary or herbal supplements. Some teens use products advertised as dietary supplements for weight loss or bodybuilding. Increasingly, products sold as dietary supplements, particularly for weight loss and bodybuilding, contain ingredients that could be harmful, including prescription drug ingredients and controlled substances. In addition, many dietary supplements haven't been tested in children. Because children's bodies aren't fully developed, the side effects of these products on children and adults may differ.

(Source: "10 Things To Know About Dietary Supplements For Children And Teens," National Center for Complementary and Integrative Health (NCCIH).)

Are There Any Risks In Taking Supplements?

Yes. Many supplements contain active ingredients that have strong biological effects in the body. This could make them unsafe in some situations and hurt or complicate your health. For example, the following actions could lead to harmful—even life-threatening—consequences.

- Combining supplements
- Using supplements with medicines (whether prescription or over-the-counter (OTC))
- Substituting supplements for prescription medicines
- Taking too much of some supplements, such as vitamin A, vitamin D, or iron

Some supplements can also have unwanted effects before, during, and after surgery. So, be sure to inform your healthcare provider, including your pharmacist about any supplements you are taking.

Some Common Dietary Supplements

- Calcium
- Echinacea
- Fish oil
- Ginseng
- Glucosamine and/or
- Chondroitin sulphate
- Garlic
- Vitamin D
- St. John's Wort
- Saw palmetto
- Ginkgo
- Green tea

Note: These examples do not represent either an endorsement or approval by FDA.

Who Is Responsible For The Safety Of Dietary Supplements?

FDA is not authorized to review dietary supplement products for safety and effectiveness before they are marketed.

The manufacturers and distributors of dietary supplements are responsible for making sure their products are safe BEFORE they go to market.

If the dietary supplement contains a NEW ingredient, manufacturers must notify FDA about that ingredient prior to marketing. However, the notification will only be reviewed by FDA (not approved) and only for safety, not effectiveness.

Manufacturers are required to produce dietary supplements in a quality manner and ensure that they do not contain contaminants or impurities, and are accurately labeled according to current Good Manufacturing Practice (cGMP) and labeling regulations.

If a serious problem associated with a dietary supplement occurs, manufacturers must report it to FDA as an adverse event. FDA can take dietary supplements off the market if they are found to be unsafe or if the claims on the products are false and misleading.

How Can I Find Out More About The Dietary Supplement I'm Taking?

Dietary supplement labels must include name and location information for the manufacturer or distributor. If you want to know more about the product that you are taking, check with the manufacturer or distributor about:

- Information to support the claims of the product
- Information on the safety and effectiveness of the ingredients in the product

How Can I Be A Smart Supplement Shopper?

Be a savvy supplement user. Here's how:

- When searching for supplements on the internet, use noncommercial sites (e.g., National Institutes of Health (NIH), FDA, U.S. Department of Agriculture (USDA)) rather than depending on information from sellers.
- If claims sound too good to be true, they probably are. Be mindful of product claims such as "works better than [a prescription drug]," "totally safe," or has "no side effects."
- Be aware that the term natural doesn't always means safe.
- Ask your healthcare provider if the supplement you're considering would be safe and beneficial for you.
- Always remember—safety first!

Making Informed Decisions And Evaluating Information

FDA, as well as health professionals and their organizations, receive many inquiries each year from consumers seeking health-related information, especially about dietary supplements. Clearly, people choosing to supplement their diets with herbals, vitamins, minerals, or other substances want to know more about the products they choose so that they can make informed decisions about them. The choice to use a dietary supplement can be a wise decision that provides health benefits. However, under certain circumstances, these products may be unnecessary for good health or they may even create unexpected risks.

Given the abundance and conflicting nature of information now available about dietary supplements, you may need help to sort the reliable information from the questionable. Below are tips and resources that we hope will help you be a savvy dietary supplement user. The principles underlying these tips are similar to those principles a savvy consumer would use for any product.

Basic Points To Consider

- **Do I need to think about my total diet?**

  Yes. Dietary supplements are intended to supplement the diets of some people, but not to replace the balance of the variety of foods important to a healthy diet. While you need enough nutrients, too much of some nutrients can cause problems.

- **Should I check with my doctor or healthcare provider before using a supplement?**

  This is a good idea, especially for certain population groups. Dietary supplements may not be risk-free under certain circumstances. If you are pregnant, nursing a baby, or have a chronic medical condition, such as, diabetes, hypertension or heart disease, be sure to consult your doctor or pharmacist before purchasing or taking any supplement. While vitamin and mineral supplements are widely used and generally considered safe for children, you may wish to check with your doctor or pharmacist before giving these or any other dietary supplements to your child. If you plan to use a dietary supplement in place of drugs or in combination with any drug, tell your healthcare provider first. Many supplements contain active ingredients that have strong biological effects and their safety is not always assured in all users. If you have certain health conditions and take these products, you may be placing yourself at risk.

- **Some supplements may interact with prescription and OTC medicines.**

  Taking a combination of supplements or using these products together with medications (whether prescription or OTC drugs) could under certain circumstances produce adverse effects, some of which could be life-threatening. Be alert to advisories about these products, whether taken alone or in combination. For example: Coumadin (a prescription medicine), *ginkgo biloba* (an herbal supplement), aspirin (an OTC drug) and vitamin E (a vitamin supplement) can each thin the blood, and taking any of these products together can increase the potential for internal bleeding. Combining St. John's Wort with certain human immunodeficiency virus (HIV) drugs significantly reduces their effectiveness. St. John's Wort may also reduce the effectiveness of prescription drugs for heart disease, depression, seizures, certain cancers or oral contraceptives.

- **Some supplements can have unwanted effects during surgery.**

  It is important to fully inform your doctor about the vitamins, minerals, herbs or any other supplements you are taking, especially before elective surgery. You may be asked to stop taking these products at least 2–3 weeks ahead of the procedure to avoid potentially dangerous supplement/drug interactions—such as changes in heart rate, blood pressure and increased bleeding—that could adversely affect the outcome of your surgery.

- **Adverse effects from the use of dietary supplements should be reported to MedWatch.**

  You, your healthcare provider, or anyone may directly to FDA if you believe it is related to the use of any dietary supplement product, by calling FDA at 800-FDA-1088 (800-332-1088), by fax at 800-FDA-0178 (800-332-0178) or reporting report a serious adverse event or illness online. FDA would like to know whenever you think a product caused you a serious problem, even if you are not sure that the product was the cause, and even if you do not visit a doctor or clinic. In addition to communicating with FDA online or by phone, you may use the MedWatch form available from the FDA website.

- **Who is responsible for ensuring the safety and efficacy of dietary supplements?**

  Under the law, manufacturers of dietary supplements are responsible for making sure their products are safe before they go to market. They are also responsible for determining that the claims on their labels are accurate and truthful. Dietary supplement products are not reviewed by the government before they are marketed, but FDA has the responsibility to take action against any unsafe dietary supplement product that reaches the market. If FDA can prove that claims on marketed dietary supplement products are false and misleading, the agency may take action also against products with such claims.

Tips On Searching The Web For Information On Dietary Supplements

When searching on the Web, try using directory sites of respected organizations, rather than doing blind searches with a search engine. Ask yourself the following questions:

- **Who operates the site?**

  Is the site run by the government, a university, or a reputable medical or health-related association (e.g., American Medical Association (AMA), American Diabetes Association, American Heart Association (AHA), National Institutes of Health, National Academies of Science (NAS), or FDA)? Is the information written or reviewed by qualified health professionals, experts in the field, academia, government, or the medical community?

- **What is the purpose of the site?**

  Is the purpose of the site to objectively educate the public or just to sell a product? Be aware of practitioners or organizations whose main interest is in marketing products, either directly or through sites with which they are linked. Commercial sites should clearly distinguish scientific information from advertisements. Most nonprofit and government sites contain no advertising; and access to the site and materials offered are usually free.

- **What is the source of the information and does it have any references?**

  Has the study been reviewed by recognized scientific experts and published in reputable peer-reviewed scientific journals, like the *New England Journal of Medicine?* Does the information say "some studies show..." or does it state where the study is listed so that you can check the authenticity of the references? For example, can the study be found in the National Library of Medicine's (NLM) database of literature citations.

- **Is the information current?**

  Check the date when the material was posted or updated. Often research or other findings are not reflected in old material, e.g., side effects or interactions with other products or new evidence that might have changed earlier thinking. Ideally, health and medical sites should be updated frequently.

- **How reliable is the Internet or e-mail solicitations?**

While the Internet is a rich source of health information, it is also an easy vehicle for spreading myths, hoaxes, and rumors about alleged news, studies, products or findings.

To avoid falling prey to such hoaxes, be skeptical and watch out for overly emphatic language with UPPERCASE LETTERS and lots of exclamation points!!!! Beware of such phrases such as: "This is not a hoax" or "Send this to everyone you know."

More Tips And To-Do's

- **Ask yourself: Does it sound too good to be true?**

  Do the claims for the product seem exaggerated or unrealistic? Are there simplistic conclusions being drawn from a complex study to sell a product? While the Web can be a valuable source of accurate, reliable information, it also has a wealth of misinformation that may not be obvious. Learn to distinguish hype from evidence-based science. Nonsensical lingo can sound very convincing. Also, be skeptical about anecdotal information from persons who have no formal training in nutrition or botanicals, or from personal testimonials (e.g., from store employees, friends, or online chat rooms and message boards) about incredible benefits or results obtained from using a product. Question these people on their training and knowledge in nutrition or medicine.

- **Think twice about chasing the latest headline.**

  Sound health advice is generally based on a body of research, not a single study. Be wary of results claiming a "quick fix" that depart from previous research and scientific beliefs. Keep in mind science does not proceed by dramatic breakthroughs, but by taking many small steps, slowly building towards a consensus. Furthermore, news stories, about the latest scientific study, especially those on TV or radio, are often too brief to include important details that may apply to you or allow you to make an informed decision.

- **Check your assumptions about the following:**

  - *1. Questionable assumption: "Even if a product may not help me, it at least won't hurt me."* It's best not to assume that this will always be true. When consumed in high enough amounts, for a long enough time, or in combination with certain other substances, all chemicals can be toxic, including nutrients, plant components, and other biologically active ingredients.

  - *2. Questionable assumption: "When I see the term 'natural,' it means that a product is healthful and safe."* Consumers can be misled if they assume this term assures wholesomeness, or that these food-like substances necessarily have milder effects, which makes them safer to use than drugs. The term "natural" on labels is not well defined and is sometimes used ambiguously to imply unsubstantiated benefits or safety. For example, many weight-loss products claim to be "natural" or "herbal" but this doesn't necessarily make them safe. Their ingredients may interact with drugs or may be dangerous for people with certain medical conditions.

- *3. Questionable assumption: "A product is safe when there is no cautionary information on the product label."* Dietary supplement manufacturers may not necessarily include warnings about potential adverse effects on the labels of their products. If consumers want to know about the safety of a specific dietary supplement, they should contact the manufacturer of that brand directly. It is the manufacturer's responsibility to determine that the supplement it produces or distributes is safe and that there is substantiated evidence that the label claims are truthful and not misleading.
- *4. Questionable assumption: "A recall of a harmful product guarantees that all such harmful products will be immediately and completely removed from the marketplace."* A product recall of a dietary supplement is voluntary and while many manufacturers do their best, a recall does not necessarily remove all harmful products from the marketplace.

- **Contact the manufacturer for more information about the specific product that you are purchasing.**

If you cannot tell whether the product you are purchasing meets the same standards as those used in the research studies you read about, check with the manufacturer or distributor. Ask to speak to someone who can address your questions, some of which may include:

1. What information does the firm have to substantiate the claims made for the product? Be aware that sometimes firms supply so-called "proof" of their claims by citing undocumented reports from satisfied consumers, or "internal" graphs and charts that could be mistaken for evidence-based research.
2. Does the firm have information to share about tests it has conducted on the safety or efficacy of the ingredients in the product?
3. Does the firm have a quality control system in place to determine if the product actually contains what is stated on the label and is free of contaminants?
4. Has the firm received any adverse events reports from consumers using their products?

Chapter 40

Botanical Products

What Is A Botanical?

A botanical is a plant or plant part valued for its medicinal or therapeutic properties, flavor, and/or scent. Herbs are a subset of botanicals. Products made from botanicals that are used to maintain or improve health may be called herbal products, botanical products, or phytomedicines.

In naming botanicals, botanists use a Latin name made up of the genus and species of the plant. Under this system the botanical black cohosh is known as *Actaea racemosa L.*, where "L" stands for Linneaus, who first described the type of plant specimen. The Office of Dietary Supplements (ODS), do not include such initials because they do not appear on most products used by consumers.

Can Botanicals Be Dietary Supplements?

To be classified as a dietary supplement, a botanical must meet the definition given below. Many botanical preparations meet the definition.

As defined by Congress in the Dietary Supplement Health and Education Act (DSHEA), which became law in 1994, a dietary supplement is a product (other than tobacco) that:

- is intended to supplement the diet;
- contains one or more dietary ingredients (including vitamins; minerals; herbs or other botanicals; amino acids; and other substances) or their constituents;

About This Chapter: This chapter includes text excerpted from "Botanical Dietary Supplements," Office of Dietary Supplements (ODS), National Institutes of Health (NIH), June 24, 2011. Reviewed January 2018.

- is intended to be taken by mouth as a pill, capsule, tablet, or liquid; and
- is labeled on the front panel as being a dietary supplement.

How Are Botanicals Commonly Sold And Prepared?

Botanicals are sold in many forms: as fresh or dried products; liquid or solid extracts; tablets, capsules, powders, tea bags, and other forms. For example, fresh ginger root is often found in the produce section of food stores; dried ginger root is sold packaged in tea bags, capsules, or tablets; and liquid preparations made from ginger root are also sold. A particular group of chemicals or a single chemical may be isolated from a botanical and sold as a dietary supplement, usually in tablet or capsule form. An example is phytoestrogens from soy products.

Common preparations include teas, decoctions, tinctures, and extracts:

- A tea, also known as an infusion, is made by adding boiling water to fresh or dried botanicals and steeping them. The tea may be drunk either hot or cold.
- Some roots, bark, and berries require more forceful treatment to extract their desired ingredients. They are simmered in boiling water for longer periods than teas, making a decoction, which also may be drunk hot or cold.
- A tincture is made by soaking a botanical in a solution of alcohol and water. Tinctures are sold as liquids and are used for concentrating and preserving a botanical. They are made in different strengths that are expressed as botanical-to-extract ratios (i.e., ratios of the weight of the dried botanical to the volume or weight of the finished product).
- An extract is made by soaking the botanical in a liquid that removes specific types of chemicals. The liquid can be used as is or evaporated to make a dry extract for use in capsules or tablets.

Phytoestrogens

Phytoestrogens are naturally occurring polycyclic phenols found in certain plants. These are chemicals that may have weak estrogenic effects when they are ingested and metabolized.

(Source: "Biomonitoring Summary—Phytoestrogens," Centers for Disease Control and Prevention (CDC).)

Are Botanical Dietary Supplements Standardized?

Standardization is a process that manufacturers may use to ensure batch-to-batch consistency of their products. In some cases, standardization involves identifying specific chemicals (also known as markers) that can be used to manufacture a consistent product. The standardization process can also provide a measure of quality control.

Dietary supplements are not required to be standardized in the United States. In fact, no legal or regulatory definition exists for standardization in the United States as it applies to botanical dietary supplements. Because of this, the term "standardization" may mean many different things. Some manufacturers use the term standardization incorrectly to refer to uniform manufacturing practices; following a recipe is not sufficient for a product to be called standardized. Therefore, the presence of the word "standardized" on a supplement label does not necessarily indicate product quality.

Ideally, the chemical markers chosen for standardization would also be the constituents that are responsible for a botanical's effect in the body. In this way, each lot of the product would have a consistent health effect. However, the components responsible for the effects of most botanicals have not been identified or clearly defined. For example, the sennosides in the botanical senna are known to be responsible for the laxative effect of the plant, but many compounds may be responsible for valerian's relaxing effect.

Are Botanical Dietary Supplements Safe?

Many people believe that products labeled "natural" are safe and good for them. This is not necessarily true because the safety of a botanical depends on many things, such as its chemical makeup, how it works in the body, how it is prepared, and the dose used.

The action of botanicals range from mild to powerful (potent). A botanical with mild action may have subtle effects. Chamomile and peppermint, both mild botanicals, are usually taken as teas to aid digestion and are generally considered safe for self-administration.

Chamomile

Chamomile is used as a dietary supplement for sleeplessness, anxiety, and gastrointestinal (GI) conditions such as upset stomach, gas, and diarrhea. It is also used topically for skin conditions and for mouth sores resulting from cancer treatment. The flowering tops of the chamomile plant are used to make teas, liquid extracts, capsules, or tablets. The herb can also be applied to the skin as a cream or an ointment, or used as a mouth rinse.

(Source: "Chamomile," National Center for Complementary and Integrative Health (NCCIH).)

Some mild botanicals may have to be taken for weeks or months before their full effects are achieved. For example, valerian may be effective as a sleep aid after 14 days of use but it is rarely effective after just one dose. In contrast a powerful botanical produces a fast result. Kava, as one example, is reported to have an immediate and powerful action affecting anxiety and muscle relaxation.

The dose and form of a botanical preparation also play important roles in its safety. Teas, tinctures, and extracts have different strengths. The same amount of a botanical may be contained in a cup of tea, a few teaspoons of tincture, or an even smaller quantity of an extract. Also, different preparations vary in the relative amounts and concentrations of chemical removed from the whole botanical. For example, peppermint tea is generally considered safe to drink but peppermint oil is much more concentrated and can be toxic if used incorrectly. It is important to follow the manufacturer's suggested directions for using a botanical and not exceed the recommended dose without the advice of a healthcare provider.

Does A Label Indicate The Quality Of A Botanical Dietary Supplement Product?

It is difficult to determine the quality of a botanical dietary supplement product from its label. The degree of quality control depends on the manufacturer, the supplier, and others in the production process.

The U.S. Food and Drug Administration (FDA) issued Good Manufacturing Practices (GMPs) for dietary supplements, a set of requirements and expectations by which dietary supplements must be manufactured, prepared, and stored to ensure quality. Manufacturers are now expected to guarantee the identity, purity, strength, and composition of their dietary supplements. For example, the GMPs aim to prevent the inclusion of the wrong ingredients, the addition of too much or too little of a dietary ingredient, the possibility of contamination (by pesticides, heavy metals such as lead, bacteria, etc.), and the improper packaging and labeling of a product.

What Methods Are Used To Evaluate The Health Benefits And Safety Of A Botanical Dietary Supplement?

Like other dietary supplements, botanicals are not required by federal law to be tested for safety and effectiveness before they are marketed, so the amount of scientific evidence available for various botanical ingredients varies widely. Some botanicals have been evaluated in scientific studies. For example, research shows that St. John's wort may be useful for short-term treatment of mild to moderate depression. Other botanical dietary supplements need more study to determine their value.

Scientists can use several approaches to evaluate botanical dietary supplements for their potential health benefits and risks. They may investigate history of use, conduct laboratory studies using cell or tissue cultures, and experiment with animals. Studies on people (e.g., individual case reports, observational studies, and clinical trials) provide the most direct evidence of a botanical supplements' effect on health and patterns of use.

Chapter 41

Herbal Medicine

An herb is a plant or plant part used for its scent, flavor, or therapeutic properties. Herbal medicines are one type of dietary supplement. They are sold as tablets, capsules, powders, teas, extracts, and fresh or dried plants. People use herbal medicines to try to maintain or improve their health.

Many people believe that products labeled "natural" are always safe and good for them. This is not necessarily true. Herbal medicines do not have to go through the testing that drugs do. Some herbs, such as comfrey and ephedra, can cause serious harm. Some herbs can interact with prescription or over-the-counter (OTC) medicines. If you are thinking about using an herbal medicine, first get information on it from reliable sources. Make sure to tell your healthcare provider about any herbal medicines you are taking.

Five Popular Herbal Medicines

1. **Evening primrose oil.** Although evening primrose oil has been used as a folk or traditional remedy for eczema, rheumatoid arthritis (RA), and menopausal symptoms, there is not enough evidence to support the use of evening primrose oil for these conditions.

About This Chapter: Text in this chapter begins with excerpts from "Herbal Medicine," MedlinePlus, National Institutes of Health (NIH), September 21, 2017; Text under the heading "Five Popular Herbal Medicines" is excerpted from "5 Tips: What You Should Know About Popular Herbs," National Center for Complementary and Integrative Health (NCCIH), September 24, 2015; Text under the heading "Six Tips: How Herbs Can Interact With Medicines" is excerpted from "6 Tips: How Herbs Can Interact With Medicines," National Center for Complementary and Integrative Health (NCCIH), September 16, 2015.

Evening primrose is a plant native to North America, but it grows in Europe and parts of the Southern hemisphere as well. It has yellow flowers that bloom in the evening. Evening primrose oil contains the fatty acid gamma-linolenic acid (GLA). Native Americans used the whole plant for bruises and its roots for hemorrhoids. The leaves were traditionally used for minor wounds, gastrointestinal (GI) complaints, and sore throats. Evening primrose oil is obtained from the seeds of the evening primrose and is usually sold in capsule form.

(Source: "Evening Primrose Oil," National Center for Complementary and Integrative Health (NCCIH).)

2. **St. John's Wort.** Study results on the effectiveness of St. John's wort for depression are conflicting. While there may be public interest in St. John's wort to treat depression, the U.S. Food and Drug Administration (FDA) has not approved its use as an OTC or prescription medicine for depression. Importantly, St. John's wort is known to affect metabolism of a number of drugs, such as antiviral medicines, antidepressants, birth control pills, and certain antiseizure medicines, and can cause serious side effects.
3. **Fenugreek.** Fenugreek is sometimes used as a folk or traditional remedy for diabetes and loss of appetite, and to stimulate milk production in breastfeeding women. However, there is not enough scientific evidence to support the use of fenugreek for these or any health condition. Given its historical use for inducing childbirth, women should use caution when taking fenugreek during pregnancy.
4. **Echinacea.** Overall, the scientific evidence on echinacea for colds is inconclusive. There is limited evidence from some studies that some echinacea preparations might reduce the length or severity of colds in adults, but results from four National Center for Complementary and Integrative Health (NCCIH)-funded clinical trials of echinacea for colds all indicated that echinacea did not reduce the length or severity of cold symptoms. Few side effects have been reported in clinical trials of echinacea, but some people may have allergic reactions.
5. **Aloe vera.** A few small studies suggest that topical aloe gel may help heal burns and abrasions. In general, topical use of aloe appears to be safe; one study, however, showed that aloe gel may inhibit healing of deep surgical wounds.

Six Tips: How Herbs Can Interact With Medicines

Many people take both dietary supplements and prescription or over-the-counter (OTC) medicines. But did you know that these medicines and supplements may interact in harmful ways? Some supplements can decrease the effects of medicines, while others can increase the effects, including unwanted side effects, of medicines. Unfortunately, for many medicines and supplements there's currently little information on possible interactions, and more research is needed. But here are six things you should know about herbs that have a high risk of potential interactions with certain medications.

1. St. John's wort interacts with many types of drugs. In most instances, it speeds up the processes that change the drug into inactive substances, leading to a decrease in drug levels in your body. However, St. John's wort can interact with some drugs, including certain types of antidepressants, and can cause harmful side effects.
2. A variety of herbs, including concentrated garlic extracts, can thin the blood in a manner similar to aspirin, which may be a problem during or after surgery.
3. Concentrated green tea supplements can interact with pseudoephedrine (a decongestant).

Tea has been used for medicinal purposes in China and Japan for thousands of years. Current uses of green tea as a beverage or dietary supplement include improving mental alertness, relieving digestive symptoms and headaches, and promoting weight loss. Green tea and its extracts, such as one of its components, epigallocatechin gallate (EGCG), have been studied for their possible protective effects against heart disease and cancer. Green tea is consumed as a beverage. It is also sold in liquid extracts, capsules, and tablets and is sometimes used in topical products (intended to be applied to the skin).

(Source: "Green Tea," National Center for Complementary and Integrative Health (NCCIH).)

4. A scientific review concluded that the herb goldenseal has a high herb-drug interaction risk with some medicines.
5. People who take medicines with a narrow therapeutic index (e.g., digoxin, cyclosporine, warfarin, and others) should take special care to tell their healthcare providers about their use of herbal supplements. A narrow therapeutic index means that if the amount of the drug is even a little too low or too high, it can cause big problems. People who take herbal supplements such as Asian ginseng, St. John's wort, and others while taking certain medicines with a narrow therapeutic index should be closely monitored.
6. When you visit your healthcare providers, it's important to tell them about all the medicines and supplements you take. Bring a written list of everything you take, how often you take them, and the doses you take.

Chapter 42

Antioxidant Supplements

Antioxidants are man-made or natural substances that may prevent or delay some types of cell damage. Diets high in vegetables and fruits, which are good sources of antioxidants, have been found to be healthy; however, research has not shown antioxidant supplements to be beneficial in preventing diseases. Examples of antioxidants include vitamins C and E, selenium, and carotenoids, such as beta-carotene, lycopene, lutein, and zeaxanthin.

About Free Radicals, Oxidative Stress, And Antioxidants

Free radicals are highly unstable molecules that are naturally formed when you exercise and when your body converts food into energy. Your body can also be exposed to free radicals from a variety of environmental sources, such as cigarette smoke, air pollution, and sunlight. Free radicals can cause "oxidative stress," a process that can trigger cell damage. Oxidative stress is thought to play a role in a variety of diseases including cancer, cardiovascular diseases, diabetes, Alzheimer disease (AD), Parkinson disease (PD), and eye diseases such as cataracts and age-related macular degeneration (AMD).

Antioxidant molecules have been shown to counteract oxidative stress in laboratory experiments (for example, in cells or animal studies). However, there is debate as to whether consuming large amounts of antioxidants in supplement form actually benefits health. There is also some concern that consuming antioxidant supplements in excessive doses may be harmful.

About This Chapter: This chapter includes text excerpted from "Antioxidants: In Depth," National Center for Complementary and Integrative Health (NCCIH), November 2013. Reviewed January 2018.

Vegetables and fruits are healthy foods and rich sources of antioxidants. Official U.S. Government policy urges people to eat more vegetables and fruits. Concerns have not been raised about the safety of any amounts of antioxidants in food.

Antioxidant Supplement Safety

- High-dose antioxidant supplements may be harmful in some cases. For example, the results of some studies have linked the use of high-dose beta-carotene supplements to an increased risk of lung cancer in smokers and use of high-dose vitamin E supplements to increased risks of hemorrhagic stroke (a type of stroke caused by bleeding in the brain) and prostate cancer.
- Like some other dietary supplements, antioxidant supplements may interact with certain medications. For example, vitamin E supplements may increase the risk of bleeding in people who are taking anticoagulant drugs ("blood thinners"). There is conflicting evidence on the effects of taking antioxidant supplements during cancer treatment; some studies suggest that this may be beneficial, but others suggest that it may be harmful. The National Cancer Institute (NCI) recommends that people who are being treated for cancer talk with their healthcare provider before taking supplements.

Should People Already Diagnosed With Cancer Take Antioxidant Supplements?

Several randomized controlled trials, some including only small numbers of patients, have investigated whether taking antioxidant supplements during cancer treatment alters the effectiveness or reduces the toxicity of specific therapies. Although these trials had mixed results, some found that people who took antioxidant supplements during cancer therapy had worse outcomes, especially if they were smokers. In some preclinical studies, antioxidants have been found to promote tumor growth and metastasis in tumor-bearing mice and to increase the ability of circulating tumor cells to metastasize. Until more is known about the effects of antioxidant supplements in cancer patients, these supplements should be used with caution.

(Source: "Antioxidants And Cancer Prevention," National Cancer Institute (NCI).)

What The Science Says

Several decades of dietary research findings suggested that consuming greater amounts of antioxidant-rich foods might help to protect against diseases. Because of these results, there has been a lot of research on antioxidant supplements. Rigorous trials of antioxidant supplements in large numbers of people have not found that high doses of antioxidant supplements prevent disease.

Observational And Laboratory Studies

Observational studies on the typical eating habits, lifestyles, and health histories of large groups of people have shown that those who ate more vegetables and fruits had lower risks of several diseases, including cardiovascular disease, stroke, cancer, and cataracts. Observational studies can provide ideas about possible relationships between dietary or lifestyle factors and disease risk, but they cannot show that one factor causes another because they cannot account for other factors that may be involved. For example, people who eat more antioxidant-rich foods might also be more likely to exercise and less likely to smoke. It may be that these factors, rather than antioxidants, account for their lower disease risk.

Researchers have also studied antioxidants in laboratory experiments. These experiments showed that antioxidants interacted with free radicals and stabilized them, thus preventing the free radicals from causing cell damage.

Clinical Trials Of Antioxidants

Because the results of such research seemed very promising, large, long-term studies—many of which were funded by the National Institutes of Health (NIH)—were conducted to test whether antioxidant supplements, when taken for periods of at least a few years, could help prevent diseases such as cardiovascular diseases and cancer in people. In these studies, volunteers were randomly assigned to take either an antioxidant or a placebo (an identical-looking product that did not contain the antioxidant). The research was conducted in a double-blind manner (neither the study participants nor the investigators knew which product was being taken). Studies of this type—called clinical trials—are designed to provide clear answers to specific questions about how a substance affects people's health.

The Age-Related Eye Disease Study (AREDS), led by the National Eye Institute (NEI) and cosponsored by other components of NIH, including National Center for Complementary and Integrative Health (NCCIH), found a beneficial effect of antioxidant supplements. This study showed that a combination of antioxidants (vitamin C, vitamin E, and beta-carotene) and zinc reduced the risk of developing the advanced stage of age-related macular degeneration (AMD) by 25 percent in people who had the intermediate stage of this disease or who had the advanced stage in only one eye. Antioxidant supplements used alone reduced the risk by about 17 percent. In the same study, however, antioxidants did not help to prevent cataracts or slow their progression.

- A follow-up study, AREDS2, found that adding omega-3 fatty acids (fish oil) to the combination of supplements did not improve its effectiveness. However, adding lutein and zeaxanthin (two carotenoids found in the eye) improved the supplement's effectiveness in people who were not taking beta-carotene and those who consumed only small amounts of lutein and zeaxanthin in foods.

Why Don't Antioxidant Supplements Work?

Most clinical studies of antioxidant supplements have not found them to provide substantial health benefits. Researchers have suggested several reasons for this, including the following:

- The beneficial health effects of a diet high in vegetables and fruits or other antioxidant-rich foods may actually be caused by other substances present in the same foods, other dietary factors, or other lifestyle choices rather than antioxidants.
- The effects of the large doses of antioxidants used in supplementation studies may be different from those of the smaller amounts of antioxidants consumed in foods.
- Differences in the chemical composition of antioxidants in foods versus those in supplements may influence their effects. For example, eight chemical forms of vitamin E are present in foods. Vitamin E supplements, on the other hand, typically include only one of these forms—alpha-tocopherol. Alpha-tocopherol also has been used in almost all research studies on vitamin E.
- For some diseases, specific antioxidants might be more effective than the ones that have been tested. For example, to prevent eye diseases, antioxidants that are present in the eye, such as lutein, might be more beneficial than those that are not found in the eye, such as beta-carotene.
- The relationship between free radicals and health may be more complex than has previously been thought. Under some circumstances, free radicals actually may be beneficial rather than harmful, and removing them may be undesirable.
- The antioxidant supplements may not have been given for a long enough time to prevent chronic diseases, such as cardiovascular diseases or cancer, which develop over decades.
- The participants in the clinical trials discussed above were either members of the general population or people who were at high risk for particular diseases. They were not

necessarily under increased oxidative stress. Antioxidants might help to prevent diseases in people who are under increased oxidative stress even if they don't prevent them in other people.

If You Are Considering Antioxidant Supplements

- Do not use antioxidant supplements to replace a healthy diet or conventional medical care, or as a reason to postpone seeing a healthcare provider about a medical problem.
- If you have AMD, consult your healthcare providers to determine whether supplements of the type used in the AREDS trial are appropriate for you.
- If you are considering a dietary supplement, first get information on it from reliable sources. Keep in mind that dietary supplements may interact with medications or other supplements and may contain ingredients not listed on the label. Your healthcare provider can advise you. If you are pregnant or nursing a child, or if you are considering giving a child a dietary supplement, it is especially important to consult your (or your child's) healthcare provider.
- Tell all of your healthcare providers about any complementary health approaches you use. Give them a full picture of what you do to manage your health. This will help ensure coordinated and safe care.

Chapter 43

Medical Marijuana

What Is Cannabis?

Cannabis, also known as marijuana, is a plant from Central Asia that is grown in many parts of the world today. The Cannabis plant produces a resin containing compounds called cannabinoids. Some cannabinoids are psychoactive (acting on the brain and changing mood or consciousness). In the United States, Cannabis is a controlled substance and has been classified as a Schedule I agent (a drug with a high potential for abuse and no currently accepted medical use).

By federal law, the possession of Cannabis (marijuana) is illegal in the United States outside of approved research settings. However, a growing number of states, territories, and the District of Columbia have enacted laws to legalize medical marijuana.

What Is Medical Marijuana?

The term medical marijuana refers to using the whole, unprocessed marijuana plant or its basic extracts to treat symptoms of illness and other conditions.

(Source: "Marijuana As Medicine," National Institute on Drug Abuse (NIDA).)

What Are Cannabinoids?

Cannabinoids are active chemicals in Cannabis that cause drug-like effects throughout the body, including the central nervous system (CNS) and the immune system. They are also

---

About This Chapter: This chapter includes text excerpted from "Cannabis And Cannabinoids (PDQ®)—Patient Version," National Cancer Institute (NCI), December 20, 2017.

known as phytocannabinoids. The main active cannabinoid in Cannabis is delta-9-THC. Another active cannabinoid is cannabidiol (CBD), which may relieve pain and lower inflammation without causing the "high" of delta-9-THC (tetrahydrocannabinols).

Cannabinoids may be useful in treating the side effects of cancer and cancer treatment.

Other possible effects of cannabinoids include:

- Anti-inflammatory activity.
- Blocking cell growth.
- Preventing the growth of blood vessels that supply tumors.
- Antiviral activity.
- Relieving muscle spasms caused by multiple sclerosis (MS).

What Is The History Of The Medical Use Of Cannabis?

The use of Cannabis for medicinal purposes dates back at least 3,000 years. It came into use in Western medicine in the 19th century and was said to relieve pain, inflammation, spasms, and convulsions.

In 1937, the U.S. Treasury began taxing Cannabis under the Marijuana Tax Act at one dollar per ounce for medicinal use and one hundred dollars per ounce for nonmedical use. The American Medical Association (AMA) opposed this regulation of Cannabis and did not want studies of its potential medicinal benefits to be limited. In 1942, Cannabis was removed from the U.S. Pharmacopoeia because of continuing concerns about its safety. In 1951, Congress passed the Boggs Act, which included Cannabis with narcotic drugs for the first time. Under the Controlled Substances Act passed by Congress in 1970, marijuana was classified as a Schedule I drug. Other Schedule I drugs include heroin, Lysergic acid diethylamide (LSD), mescaline, methaqualone, and gamma-hydroxybutyrate (GHB).

Although Cannabis was not believed to have any medicinal use, the U.S. government distributed it to patients on a case-by-case basis under the Compassionate Use Investigational New Drug (IND) program started in 1978. This program was closed to new patients in 1992.

Researchers have studied how cannabinoids act on the brain and other parts of the body. Cannabinoid receptors (molecules that bind cannabinoids) have been discovered in brain cells and nerve cells in other parts of the body. The presence of cannabinoid receptors on immune system cells suggests that cannabinoids may have a role in immunity.

Nabiximols (Sativex) is a Cannabis extract that contains delta-9-THC and cannabidiol (CBD). Nabiximols is approved in Canada (under the Notice of Compliance with Conditions) for relief of pain in patients with advanced cancer or multiple sclerosis.

If Cannabis Is Illegal, How Do Some Cancer Patients In The United States Use It?

Though federal law prohibits the use of Cannabis, the map below shows the states and territories that have legalized Cannabis for medical purposes. Some other states have legalized only one ingredient in Cannabis, such as cannabidiol (CBD), and these states are not included in the map. Medical marijuana laws vary from state to state.

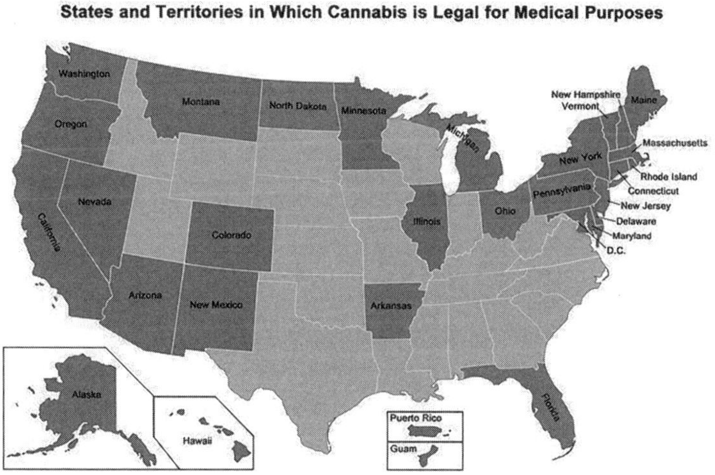

States and Territories in Which Cannabis is Legal for Medical Purposes

Figure 43.1. Medical Use Of Cannabis In The United States

How Is Cannabis Administered?

Cannabis may be taken by mouth or may be inhaled. When taken by mouth (in baked products or as an herbal tea), the main psychoactive ingredient in Cannabis (delta-9-THC) is processed by the liver, making an additional psychoactive chemical.

When Cannabis is smoked and inhaled, cannabinoids quickly enter the bloodstream. The additional psychoactive chemical is produced in smaller amounts than when taken by mouth.

A growing number of clinical trials are studying a medicine made from an extract of Cannabis that contains specific amounts of cannabinoids. This medicine is sprayed under the tongue.

Have Any Preclinical (Laboratory Or Animal) Studies Been Conducted Using Cannabis Or Cannabinoids?

Preclinical studies of cannabinoids have investigated the following:

Antitumor Activity

- Studies in mice and rats have shown that cannabinoids may inhibit tumor growth by causing cell death, blocking cell growth, and blocking the development of blood vessels needed by tumors to grow. Laboratory and animal studies have shown that cannabinoids may be able to kill cancer cells while protecting normal cells.
- A study in mice showed that cannabinoids may protect against inflammation of the colon and may have potential in reducing the risk of colon cancer, and possibly in its treatment.
- A laboratory study of delta-9-THC in hepatocellular carcinoma (liver cancer) cells showed that it damaged or killed the cancer cells. The same study of delta-9-THC in mouse models of liver cancer showed that it had antitumor effects. Delta-9-THC has been shown to cause these effects by acting on molecules that may also be found in nonsmall cell lung cancer cells and breast cancer cells.
- A laboratory study of cannabidiol (CBD) in estrogen receptor positive and estrogen receptor negative breast cancer cells showed that it caused cancer cell death while having little effect on normal breast cells. Studies in mouse models of metastatic breast cancer showed that cannabinoids may lessen the growth, number, and spread of tumors.
- A review of 34 studies of cannabinoids in glioma tumor models found that all but one study showed that cannabinoids can kill cancer cells without harming normal cells.
- A laboratory study of cannabidiol (CBD) in human glioma cells showed that when given along with chemotherapy, CBD may make chemotherapy more effective and increase cancer cell death without harming normal cells. Studies in mouse models of cancer showed that CBD together with delta-9-THC may make chemotherapy such as temozolomide more effective.

Stimulating Appetite

- Many animal studies have shown that delta-9-THC and other cannabinoids stimulate appetite and can increase food intake.

Pain Relief

- Cannabinoid receptors (molecules that bind cannabinoids) have been studied in the brain, spinal cord, and nerve endings throughout the body of animals to understand their roles in pain relief.
- Cannabinoids have been studied for anti-inflammatory effects that may play a role in pain relief.
- Animal studies have shown that cannabinoids may prevent nerve problems (pain, numbness, tingling, swelling, and muscle weakness) caused by some types of chemotherapy.

Nausea And Vomiting

- Cannabinoid receptors found in brain cells may have a role in controlling nausea and vomiting. Animal studies have shown that delta-9-THC and other cannabinoids may act on cannabinoid receptors to prevent vomiting caused by certain types of chemotherapy.

Anxiety And Sleep

- Cannabinoid receptors found in the brain and other parts of the nervous system may be involved in controlling mood and anxiety.
- Antianxiety effects of cannabidiol (CBD) have been shown in several animal models.

Have Any Side Effects Or Risks Been Reported From Cannabis And Cannabinoids?

Adverse side effects of cannabinoids may include:

- Rapid beating of the heart.
- Low blood pressure.
- Muscle relaxation.
- Bloodshot eyes.
- Slowed digestion and movement of food by the stomach and intestines.
- Dizziness.
- Depression.

- Hallucinations.
- Paranoia.

Because Cannabis smoke contains many of the same substances as tobacco smoke, there are concerns about how inhaled cannabis affects the lungs. A study of over 5,000 men and women without cancer over a period of 20 years found that smoking tobacco was linked with some loss of lung function but that occasional and low use of cannabis was not linked with loss of lung function.

Because use of Cannabis over a long time may have harmful effects on the endocrine and reproductive systems, rates of testicular germ cell tumors (TGCTs) in Cannabis users have been studied. Larger studies that follow patients over time and laboratory studies of cannabinoid receptors in TGCTs are needed to find if there is a link between Cannabis use and a higher risk of TGCTs.

A review of bladder cancer rates in Cannabis users and nonusers was done in over 84,000 men who took part in the California Men's Health Study. Over 16 years of follow-up and adjusting for age, race/ethnic group and body mass index (BMI), rates of bladder cancer were found to be 45 percent lower in Cannabis users than in men who did not report Cannabis use.

Both Cannabis and cannabinoids may be addictive.

Symptoms of withdrawal from cannabinoids may include:

- Irritability.
- Trouble sleeping.
- Restlessness.
- Hot flashes.
- Nausea and cramping (rarely occur).

These symptoms are mild compared to withdrawal from opiates and usually lessen after a few days.

Are Cannabis Or Cannabinoids Approved By The U.S. Food And Drug Administration For Use As A Cancer Treatment In The United States?

The U.S. Food and Drug Administration (FDA) has not approved Cannabis or cannabinoids for use as a cancer treatment.

Are Cannabis Or Cannabinoids Approved By The U.S. Food and Drug Administration For Use As A Treatment For Cancer-Related Symptoms Or Side Effects Of Cancer Therapy?

Cannabis is not approved by the U.S. Food and Drug Administration (FDA) for the treatment of any cancer-related symptom or side effect of cancer therapy.

Two cannabinoids (dronabinol and nabilone) are approved by the FDA for the treatment of chemotherapy-related nausea and vomiting in patients who have not responded to standard therapy.

Point To Remember

The FDA has approved two pill versions of THC to treat nausea in cancer chemotherapy patients and to stimulate appetite in some patients with AIDS. Also, a new product that is a chemically controlled mixture of THC and cannabidiol (another chemical found in the marijuana plant) is available in several countries outside the United States as a mouth spray. However, it's important to remember that because marijuana is usually smoked into the lungs and has ingredients that can vary from plant to plant, its health risks may outweigh its value as a treatment. Scientists continue to investigate safe ways that patients can use THC and other marijuana ingredients as medicine.

(Source: "Marijuana: Facts For Teens—Want To Know More? Some FAQs About Marijuana," National Institute on Drug Abuse (NIDA).)

Chapter 44

Popular Fad Diets

Introduction To Popular Fad Diets

The many popular diets and diet plans on the market today can be confusing and overwhelming for consumers to navigate. People who want to lose weight are bombarded with advertisements for various diets all claiming to provide the secret to rapid weight loss with little or no effort. Some of these diets eliminate or restrict various foods, while others focus on including only certain foods. A diet can be considered a fad if it promises to deliver drastic weight loss in a short amount of time, without exercise, and if it is based on an unbalanced approach to nutrition. Many popular fad diets can be organized by type: high protein, low carbohydrate, fasting, food-specific, liquid only, and so on.

High-Protein Diets

High-protein diets promote an eating plan based largely on foods containing protein, usually meat, eggs, cheese, and other dairy products. The theory behind high-protein diets is that the body must work harder to digest protein, and in doing so, more calories are burned. Studies have found that diets high in protein can cause certain health problems, as the body works to process excess protein. High-protein diets can cause rapid initial weight loss as the body eliminates water while processing extra protein. Typically, any weight lost on a high-protein diet will be regained.

About This Chapter: "Popular Fad Diets," © 2015 Omnigraphics. Reviewed January 2018.

Low-Carbohydrate Diets

The main premise of low-carbohydrate diets is the severe restriction of calories from carbohydrates (sugar). Most low-carbohydrate diets suggest replacing foods high in carbohydrates with foods high in protein. In this way, low-carbohydrate diets are similar to high-protein diets. A low-carbohydrate diet is often high in fat. A high-fat diet causes a condition known as ketosis, which can act as an appetite suppressant. The theory of low-carbohydrate diets is that the suppressed appetite will result in the dieter consuming fewer calories overall. Studies of low-carbohydrate diets have shown that dieters are at risk for health problems including kidney malfunction and heart disease. Many people who follow a low-carbohydrate diet report feeling sluggish and tired, and typically any weight that is lost will be regained.

Detoxifying Diets

Detoxifying diets are often high-fiber diets, and sometimes include increased consumption of fats and oils. The theory of this type of detoxification is that the fiber helps the dieter to feel full, therefore consuming fewer calories throughout the day. It is also believed that a high-fiber diet will cleanse the digestive system through the elimination of more solid waste. Side effects of a high-fiber detoxifying diet often include gastrointestinal distress, bloating, cramps, and dehydration. Studies have shown no permanent weight loss from this type of detoxifying diet.

Fasting Diets

Fasting diets require dieters to consume nothing but clear liquids for a short period of time, typically one to five days. This is believed to help rid the body of toxins. Fasting can result in temporary weight loss due to consuming far fewer calories than normal, though the weight generally returns once the fast is ended. Fasting produces a host of side effects, including dizziness, lethargy, and feeling weak or tired.

Food-Specific Diets

Food-specific diets recommend consumption of a single type of food, such as grapefruit, cabbage or protein shakes. These diets are based on the theory that certain foods have special properties that promote weight-loss. Food-specific diets do not provide the range of vitamins, minerals, and other nutrients needed to support bodily functions. If maintained over an extended period of time, the side effects of food-specific diets can be serious.

Popular Diet Plans

The Atkins Diet

The Atkins Diet is a low-carbohydrate, high-protein diet created by Dr. Robert Atkins, an American cardiologist. The main premise of the Atkins Diet is that eating too many carbohydrates causes obesity and other health problems. A diet that is low in carbohydrates produces metabolic activity that results in less hunger and also in weight loss. The Atkins Diet is structured in four phases: induction; weight loss; pre-maintenance; lifetime maintenance. Dieters move through the four phases at their own pace. Early phases of the Atkins Diet allow consumption of seafood, poultry, meat, eggs, cheese, salad vegetables, oils, butter, and cream. Later phases allow consumption of foods such as nuts, fruits, wine, beans, whole grains, and other vegetables. The Atkins Diet recommends avoidance of certain foods such as fruit, bread, most grains, starchy vegetables, and dairy products other than cheese, cream, and butter. The Atkins Diet may help people feel full longer, and may result in weight loss as long as the diet in continued. Side effects may result from consuming low amounts of fiber and certain vitamins and minerals, while consuming larger amounts of saturated fat, cholesterol, and red meat.

The Zone Diet

The Zone Diet was created by Dr. Barry Spears and is based on the genetic evolution of humans. The main premise of the Zone Diet is that humans should maintain a diet similar to that of our ancient hunter-gatherer ancestors. The Zone Diet focuses on lean protein, natural carbohydrates (fruit) and natural fiber (vegetables) while avoiding or eliminating processed carbohydrates such as grains and products made from grains. The Zone Diet recommends a food plan that is made up of 40 percent natural carbohydrates. 30 percent fat, and 30 percent protein. The emphasis is on food choices, not amount of calories. This percentage should apply to every meal and snack that is eaten. Close evaluation of the Zone Diet has revealed that at its core, the Zone Diet is a very low-calorie eating plan that is lacking in certain nutrients, vitamins, and minerals.

Weight Watchers

Weight Watchers was founded by Jean Nidetch in 1963. The Weight Watchers program focuses on weight loss through diet, exercise, and the use of support networks. Members are given the option of joining a group or following the program online. In either case, educational materials and support are available to assist members. The Weight Watchers support network is considered a critical aspect of the program, as it is believed that dieters need constant positive reinforcement in order to achieve and maintain long-term weight loss. The Weight Watchers program is structured in two phases: weight loss and maintenance. During weight loss, dieters work to lose weight slowly, with the goal of one to two pounds per week. Once the goal weight has been attained, dieters move into the maintenance phase, during which they gradually adjust their food intake until they are neither losing nor gaining weight. In general, Weight Watchers is viewed as providing a healthy approach to dieting.

Ornish Lifestyle Medicine

The Ornish Lifestyle Medicine program was created by Dr. Dean Ornish. The main premise of the program is that foods are neither good nor bad, but some are healthier than others. The Ornish diet focuses on fruits, vegetables, whole grains, legumes, soy products, nonfat dairy, natural egg whites, and fats that contain omega three fatty acids. The Ornish diet is plant-based; meat, poultry, and fish are excluded. Portion control is recommended, but caloric intake is not restricted unless a person is trying to lose weight. The program recommends small, frequent meals spread out throughout the day to support constant energy and avoid hunger. The consumption of caffeine is discouraged though allowed in small amounts. The Ornish program recommends exercise and low-dose multivitamin supplements. In general, the Ornish program is viewed as a healthy diet.

Diet Safety

Fad diets may produce initial weight loss results, but the potential for undesirable side effects should not be ignored. The human body needs simple carbohydrates (glucose) for energy and brain function. Low-carbohydrate and high-protein diets are not nutritionally balanced enough to meet the needs of children and some adults, particularly women who are pregnant, plan to become pregnant, or are nursing a baby. If maintained for an extended period of time, high-protein, low-carbohydrate diets can result in health problems such as heart disease, kidney problems, and certain cancers.

Weight loss is achieved by eating fewer calories than are consumed by physical activity. Because most fad diets require people to consumer very few calories, these diets can result in weight loss. However, because most fad diets are not nutritionally balanced and cannot be maintained for long periods of time, people usually find that any weight lost is regained once they stop following the diet and return to their old eating habits. The most effective weight-loss strategies are those that include a healthy, balanced diet combined with exercise.

References

1. "Diet Fads vs. Diet Truths," January 2004.
2. Nordqvist, Christian. "The Eight Most Popular Diets Today," Medical News Today, October 1, 2015.
3. "Nutrition Fact Sheet," Alaska Department of State Health Services, Nutrition Services Section, 2005.

Chapter 45

Oral Probiotics

What Are Probiotics?

Probiotics are live microorganisms that are intended to have health benefits. Products sold as probiotics include foods (such as yogurt), dietary supplements, and products that aren't used orally, such as skin creams.

Although people often think of bacteria and other microorganisms as harmful "germs," many microorganisms help our bodies function properly. For example, bacteria that are normally present in our intestines help digest food, destroy disease-causing microorganisms, and produce vitamins. Large numbers of microorganisms live on and in our bodies. In fact, microorganisms in the human body outnumber human cells by 10 to 1. Many of the microorganisms in probiotic products are the same as or similar to microorganisms that naturally live in our bodies.

The History Of Probiotics

The concept behind probiotics was introduced in the early 20th century, when Nobel laureate Elie Metchnikoff, known as the "father of probiotics," proposed that consuming beneficial microorganisms could improve people's health. Researchers continued to investigate this idea, and the term "probiotics"—meaning "for life"—eventually came into use.

What Kinds Of Microorganisms Are In Probiotics?

Probiotics may contain a variety of microorganisms. The most common are bacteria that belong to groups called *Lactobacillus* and *Bifidobacterium*. Each of these two broad groups

About This Chapter: This chapter includes text excerpted from "Probiotics: In Depth," National Center for Complementary and Integrative Health (NCCIH), October 2016.

includes many types of bacteria. Other bacteria may also be used as probiotics, and so may yeasts such as *Saccharomyces boulardii.*

Probiotics, Prebiotics, And Synbiotics

Prebiotics are not the same as probiotics. The term "prebiotics" refers to dietary substances that favor the growth of beneficial bacteria over harmful ones. The term "synbiotics" refers to products that combine probiotics and prebiotics.

What The Science Says About The Effectiveness Of Probiotics

Researchers have studied probiotics to find out whether they might help prevent or treat a variety of health problems, including:

- Digestive disorders such as diarrhea caused by infections, antibiotic-associated diarrhea (AAD), irritable bowel syndrome (IBS), and inflammatory bowel disease (IBD)
- Allergic disorders such as atopic dermatitis (AD) (eczema) and allergic rhinitis (hay fever)
- Tooth decay, periodontal disease, and other oral health problems
- Colic in infants
- Liver disease
- The common cold
- Prevention of necrotizing enterocolitis in very low birth weight infants

There's preliminary evidence that some probiotics are helpful in preventing diarrhea caused by infections and antibiotics and in improving symptoms of irritable bowel syndrome, but more needs to be learned. We still don't know which probiotics are helpful and which are not. We also don't know how much of the probiotic people would have to take or who would most likely benefit from taking probiotics. Even for the conditions that have been studied the most, researchers are still working toward finding the answers to these questions.

For Better Gut Health

Consider probiotics. Talk with your doctor about taking probiotics (supplemental healthful bacteria). They may ease constipation and IBS symptoms.

(Source: "Keeping Your Gut In Check," NIH News in Health, *National Institutes of Health (NIH).)*

Probiotics are not all alike. For example, if a specific kind of *Lactobacillus* helps prevent an illness, that doesn't necessarily mean that another kind of *Lactobacillus* would have the same effect or that any of the *Bifidobacterium* probiotics would do the same thing.

Although some probiotics have shown promise in research studies, strong scientific evidence to support specific uses of probiotics for most health conditions is lacking. The U.S. Food and Drug Administration (FDA) has not approved any probiotics for preventing or treating any health problem. Some experts have cautioned that the rapid growth in marketing and use of probiotics may have outpaced scientific research for many of their proposed uses and benefits.

How Might Probiotics Work?

Probiotics may have a variety of effects in the body, and different probiotics may act in different ways.

Probiotics might:

- Help to maintain a desirable community of microorganisms
- Stabilize the digestive tract's barriers against undesirable microorganisms or produce substances that inhibit their growth
- Help the community of microorganisms in the digestive tract return to normal after being disturbed (for example, by an antibiotic or a disease)
- Outcompete undesirable microorganisms
- Stimulate the immune response

What The Science Says About The Safety And Side Effects Of Probiotics

Whether probiotics are likely to be safe for you depends on the state of your health.

In people who are generally healthy, probiotics have a good safety record. Side effects, if they occur at all, usually consist only of mild digestive symptoms such as gas.

On the other hand, there have been reports linking probiotics to severe side effects, such as dangerous infections, in people with serious underlying medical problems. The people who are most at risk of severe side effects include critically ill patients, those who have had surgery, very sick infants, and people with weakened immune systems

Even for healthy people, there are uncertainties about the safety of probiotics. Because many research studies on probiotics haven't looked closely at safety, there isn't enough information right now to answer some safety questions. Most of our knowledge about safety comes from studies of *Lactobacillus* and *Bifidobacterium*; less is known about other probiotics. Information on the long-term safety of probiotics is limited, and safety may differ from one type of probiotic to another. For example, even though a National Center for Complementary and Integrative Health (NCCIH)-funded study showed that a particular kind of *Lactobacillus* appears safe in healthy adults age 65 and older, this does not mean that all probiotics would necessarily be safe for people in this age group.

Quality Concerns About Probiotic Products

Some probiotic products have been found to contain smaller numbers of live microorganisms than expected. In addition, some products have been found to contain bacterial strains other than those listed on the label.

Chapter 46

Enzyme Therapy

What Are Enzymes?

Enzymes, or biological catalysts, are proteins that speed up chemical reactions in living organisms. Biological catalysts are prepared from renewable materials, operate near room temperature and atmospheric pressure, in water at neutral pH, and can be evolved in the laboratory using the modern methods of molecular biology to be more active, more selective or longer-lived.

Because enzymes are highly specific, more direct synthetic routes to desired molecules can be conceived, and as a result, less waste is produced in the course of producing those molecules. In the biosynthetic pathway to the creation of cholesterol, for instance, there are more than 50 different chemical bonds present—many of them almost identical to each other—and an enzyme would cause a reaction to occur at just one of those bonds.

Enzymes In Digestion

The digestive system carries out both physical and chemical digestion. Physical digestion, like chewing, breaks food into smaller particles, increasing the surface area. Chemical digestion

About This Chapter: Text under the heading "What Are Enzymes?" is excerpted from "On The Path Toward Bionic Enzymes," U.S. Department of Energy (DOE), June 15, 2016; Text under the heading "Enzymes In Digestion" is excerpted from "Digestive Enzyme Lab (Spit Lab)," U.S. Department of Energy (DOE), June 15, 2009. Reviewed January 2018; Text beginning with the heading "Enzyme Replacement Therapy" is excerpted from "Drug Record: Enzyme Replacement Therapy," LiverTox®, National Institutes of Health (NIH), March 10, 2016; Text beginning with the heading "Pancreatic Enzyme Products" is excerpted from "Updated Questions And Answers For Healthcare Professionals And The Public: Use An Approved Pancreatic Enzyme Product (PEP)," U.S. Food and Drug Administration (FDA), October 20, 2016.

breaks macromolecules into their monomers so they can be transported via the circulatory and lymphatic system to the rest of the body. Chemical digestion is dependent on the use of enzymes to catalyze reactions by lowering the activation energy necessary for those reactions to take place. Enzymes are specific and that is equally true for digestive enzymes.

The first digestive enzyme that food encounters on its trip through the body is alpha amylase, in the mouth. Alpha amylase begins carbohydrate digestion by breaking starch into maltose units (two units of glucose bonded together). Alpha amylase works at an optimal pH of 7 and a body temp of 36.99°C. This enzyme will be quickly denatured when it reaches the stomach with a pH of 2. Carbohydrate digestion will resume in the small intestine with different carbohydrases produced by the pancreas and the small intestine.

Enzymes are critical to the functioning of the digestive system. If an enzyme is missing or in deficient supply, it can cause lots of problems. This is the case for many people that are lactose intolerant. They lack or have a very low level of an enzyme called lactase. Lactase is normally produced by the small intestine and it breaks down the disaccharide lactose, also known as milk sugar, into glucose and galactose (another monosaccharide similar to glucose). Without this enzyme, many people experience abdominal cramps, bloating, and diarrhea when they consume dairy products.

There are two main types of lactose intolerance. The first type, primary lactose intolerance, usually begins around the age of 2 and is progressive. Many do not experience symptoms until their late teens or early 20s. This type of lactose intolerance appears to be genetic, showing up with greater frequency in certain ethnic groups. Secondary lactose intolerance is caused by injury to the small intestine. It may occur due to severe diarrheal infection or chemotherapy. There is no genetic connection with secondary lactose intolerance and it can occur at any age.

Enzyme Replacement Therapy

Enzyme replacement therapy (ERT) refers to treatment of congenital enzyme deficiencies using purified human, animal or recombinant enzyme preparations. The enzymes are given parenterally, usually by intravenous infusion. The diseases treated are generally rare genetic disorders which lead to severe disability and premature death.

Indications For ERT

Enzyme replacement therapy is typically used to replace a missing or deficient enzyme in a person with an inherited enzyme deficiency syndrome. The missing enzyme is replaced by infusions of an enzyme that is purified from human or animal tissue or blood or produced by novel recombinant techniques. Typically, the enzyme is modified to allow for a longer half-life, more potent activity, resistance to degradation or targeting to a specific organ, tissue or cell type. The first successful enzyme replacement therapies were for alpha-1-antitrypsin (A1AT) deficiency using plasma derived purified human A1AT. A1AT deficiency is associated with early onset emphysema attributed to the lack of leukocyte elastase inhibitor which leads to progressive pulmonary damage. Small prospective studies suggested a benefit from augmentation therapy, raising the levels of A1AT in serum by infusing the enzyme purified from human serum. This therapy was eventually shown to be beneficial, particularly in patients with early or intermediate pulmonary dysfunction and was quite safe, without the occurrence of viral hepatitis, despite being prepared from human plasma.

A second form of successful enzyme replacement therapy was established for Gaucher disease, an inherited deficiency of lysosomal acid β-glucocerebrosidase that leads to accumulation of the substrate (glucocerebroside and its other breakdown products such as ceramide) in lysosomes. The major tissues affected are liver, spleen and bone. The glucocerebrosidase was initially prepared from placental tissue and was modified to allow its specific uptake by macrophages and delivery into lysosomes. Subsequently, recombinant forms of glucocerebrosidase have been developed and now constitute the standard of care for type 1 Gaucher disease.

Subsequently, similar or related approaches have been taken to treat other enzyme deficiency syndromes such as adenosine deaminase deficiency, lysosomal acid lipase deficiency, Fabry disease, Pompe disease, Hurler and Hunter syndrome and several of the rarer forms of mucopolysaccharidoses.

Adverse Effects Of ERT

Natural purified and recombinant enzymes are generally well tolerated with minimal systemic adverse reactions. The usual major reactions to enzyme replacement therapy are local infusion reactions and hypersensitivity reactions. Hypersensitivity can be a difficult problem, not just in causing allergic symptoms but also in causing inactivity of the enzyme by cross reacting antibodies. Hypersensitivity reactions are generally more common and more severe in patients with total absence of the enzyme, rather than a deficiency or minor amino acid mutation that inactivates the protein. Hypersensitivity reactions can be severe with rash, fever, hypotension, angioneurotic edema, bronchospasm, anaphylaxis and cardiopulmonary collapse. Most reactions, however, are mild and transient and may be prevented by premedication with antihistamines, antipyretics or corticosteroids.

Pancreatic Enzyme Products

Pancreatic enzyme products (PEPs) contain the active ingredient pancrelipase, a mixture of the digestive enzymes amylase, lipase, and protease. These digestive enzymes are used to improve food digestion in patients whose bodies do not produce enough pancreatic enzymes. PEPs have been used to treat patients with various pancreatic disorders, including cystic fibrosis, Shwachman-Diamond syndrome, chronic pancreatitis, pancreatic tumors, or removal of all or a part of the pancreas. Although PEPs have been used for several decades, they have been marketed in the United States as unapproved products.

Why Has Food And Drug Administration (FDA) Been Concerned About The PEPs That Are Not Approved?

Several years ago, FDA became aware that unapproved PEPs contained variable amounts of the therapeutic enzymes (lipase, amylase, and protease), which were causing patients to notice changes in their ability to digest food due to underdosing, or adverse events due to overdosing. An important characteristic of the drug approval process is that companies must demonstrate they are able to manufacture their products with sufficient consistency and quality to ensure patients do not experience problems due to dose variation.

Which PEPs Are Approved By The FDA?

As of May 17, 2012, FDA has approved six PEPs because they meet the regulatory standards for quality, safety, and effectiveness. Creon and Zenpep were approved for marketing in 2009, Pancreaze was approved in April 2010, Ultresa and Viokace were approved in March 2012 and Pertzye was approved May 17, 2012. All approved PEP products have drug labels with important information for healthcare professionals and Medication Guides for patients that explain the product's risks and benefits.

Chapter 47

Detoxification Diets

Detoxification is concerned with identifying and eliminating toxic substances that may accumulate in the human body. It is a common technique used in alternative medicine for the purpose of curing disease and improving general health. Detoxification has been used for centuries by practitioners of the Ayurvedic and Chinese medical systems, who have taught that eating certain types of food can help eliminate toxins from the body and restore good health. Complementary and alternative medicine (CAM) practitioners often recommend detoxification therapies for people with allergies, anxiety, asthma, cancer, depression, diabetes, headaches, heart disease, obesity, and other chronic conditions. People who are exposed to high levels of toxic substances in the environment due to industrial accidents or pollution may also benefit from detoxification therapy.

Detoxification programs have increased in popularity in recent years. The trend may have started with celebrities touting the benefits of various regimens designed to cleanse the body of chemicals and impurities, cure chronic illnesses, promote weight loss, or end addictions. Such programs have quickly gained adherents among ordinary people hoping to reverse the ill effects of fast food, sugar, caffeine, and other dietary excesses. Detoxification has emerged as a major nutrition and health industry worldwide, with hundreds of different diets, supplements, and holiday retreats promising to help people cleanse their bodies of toxins. The options range from simple diets based on cucumber or grapefruit juice to elaborate vacation packages offering fasts, mud baths, and colonic irrigation. Many people sign up for detoxification therapies as inpatients in order to speed up the process and gain the reassurance of having a practitioner monitor their treatment.

The Idea Behind Detoxification

From pollution in the air to pesticides on crops and growth hormones in meat, people are exposed to a wide variety of organic pollutants and chemical contaminants every day. While the human body naturally eliminates many harmful substances in wastes, some toxic substances can buildup in fat cells and other living tissues. Heavy metals, persistent organic pollutants, and fat-soluble chemicals, for instance, tend to bioaccumulate and remain in the body's cells for a long time. The buildup of toxins can contribute to serious physiological problems, including cancer and diseases of the kidneys, liver, lungs, and heart. Detoxification programs attempt to address these problems by ridding the body of toxins that pose health risks. Detoxification thus holds an obvious appeal for many people. They like the idea that following a special diet can remove harmful substances from the body and eliminate the health risks associated with them.

The Science Behind Detoxification

The mainstream medical community, however, tends to regard detoxification as a myth. Although toxins are undoubtedly present in the environment, they argue that the body is capable of eliminating those encountered by a typical person through natural mechanisms involving the skin, lungs, liver, and kidneys. If a person is exposed to such high levels of toxic substances that their bodily systems cannot process and eliminate them, then they are likely to require medical attention. Critics say that there is no scientific evidence to substantiate the lofty claims made by promoters of various detoxification programs. They argue that no special diet, supplement, or regimen can eliminate all toxins from the body, and that most of these programs are unlikely to lead to significant improvements in health. Critics point out that the makers of detoxification products—ranging from smoothies to shampoos—do not specify exactly what toxins the products purportedly eliminate. As a result, a patient's bodily levels of these toxins cannot be measured before and after they undergo treatment in order to prove the products' efficacy. The only kind of medically validated detoxification programs are those intended to help people overcome alcohol or drug addictions.

Types Of Detoxification Programs

Although there are many different detoxification diets and programs available, most are based on the same principles. They encourage people to restrict their exposure to chemicals for a specific period of time (usually 5–7 days) while also consuming foods or supplements that are believed to stimulate the release of stored toxins from the body. Many detoxification diets begin with a period of fasting, which is intended to rest the organs and reset the digestive system. Ancient Chinese and Ayurvedic medical traditions claim that regular fasting cleanses the digestive tract and enhances health and longevity.

Rather than restricting food intake in general, other detoxification diets focus on eliminating certain foods that are believed to increase the toxin load in the body—such alcohol, caffeine, refined sugar, saturated fats, and processed grains. Along the same lines, some detoxification programs recommend minimizing exposure to household cleaners, personal care products, lawn treatments, and other common environmental sources of toxic chemicals, and replacing them with natural alternatives when possible.

After reducing the exposure to toxins, the next step in many detoxification programs involves stimulating the body to eliminate built-up toxins from the organs and tissues. Common strategies for achieving this goal include drinking lots of water to improve kidney function, eating foods high in fiber to improve colon function, exercising to increase blood circulation, sitting in a sauna to excrete toxins through sweating, getting a massage to release toxins in muscles and fat tissues, and exfoliating to remove dead skin.

Finally, many detoxification programs recommend refuelling the body with healthy nutrients. Although countless detox diet plans exist, most tend to emphasize a high-fiber diet full of organic fruits and vegetables and lots of water. Some programs promote the use of dietary supplements to aid in the detoxification process. Many of these supplements are diuretics or laxatives made from herbal extracts. They should be used with care, as diuretics can cause dehydration and fatigue, while laxatives can lead to frequent bowel movements and malabsorption of nutrients.

The Pros And Cons Of Detoxification

Despite the disapproval of the mainstream medical community, millions of people try detoxification programs each year, and some of them swear that they lose weight, feel better, or experience other health benefits. Some aspects of the typical detox diet can lead to healthier food choices and more mindful eating. Many people abstain from alcohol, tobacco, and caffeine during detoxification, for instance, and increase their consumption of fruits, vegetables, whole grains, and water. Completing a detoxification program can help people break bad eating habits by retraining the palate to enjoy whole foods and reject processed foods. It can also help people recover from disorders like emotional eating or binge eating.

By temporarily limiting food choices, detox diets can also help people consume fewer calories and lose weight. In many cases, though, the weight loss takes the form of water and stored glycogen, and people will typically regain the pounds once they resume a normal eating pattern. The restrictions in some detoxification plans can also create nutritional deficiencies, especially for teenagers, pregnant or lactating women, or people with health conditions like diabetes or cardiovascular disease. Doctors warn that detox diets—and especially those that involve fasting—can be harmful to the health and well-being of these groups of people. Finally, detoxification programs and supplements can be very expensive.

References

1. Smith, Deborahann. "10 Ways To Detoxify Your Body," Gaiam Life, 2014.
2. Torrens, Kerry. "What Is A Detox Diet?" BBC GoodFood, n.d.

Chapter 48

What You Need To Know About Gerson Therapy

What Is The Gerson Therapy?

The Gerson therapy has been used by some people to treat cancer and other diseases. It is based on the role of minerals, enzymes, and other dietary factors. There are 3 key parts to the therapy:

- **Diet.** Organic fruits, vegetables, and whole grains to give the body plenty of vitamins, minerals, enzymes, and other nutrients. The fruits and vegetables are low in sodium (salt) and high in potassium.
- **Supplementation.** The addition of certain substances to the diet to help correct cell metabolism (the chemical changes that take place in a cell to make energy and basic materials needed for the body's life processes).
- **Detoxification.** Treatments, including enemas, to remove toxic (harmful) substances from the body.

Detox Programs

Detox programs may involve a variety of approaches, such as:

- Fasting
- Consuming only juices or other liquids for several days

About This Chapter: This chapter includes text excerpted from "Gerson Therapy (PDQ®)—Patient Version," National Cancer Institute (NCI), January 7, 2015.

- Eating a very restricted selection of foods
- Using various dietary supplements or other commercial products
- Cleansing the colon (lower intestinal tract) with enemas, laxatives, or colon hydrotherapy (also called "colonic irrigation" or "colonics")
- Combining some of these or other approaches.

(Source: "Detoxes And Cleanses," National Center for Complementary and Integrative Health (NCCIH).)

What Is The History Of The Discovery And Use Of The Gerson Therapy As A Complementary Or Alternative Treatment For Cancer?

The Gerson therapy was named after Dr. Max B. Gerson (1881–1959), who first used it to treat his migraine headaches. In the 1930's, Dr. Gerson's therapy became known to the public as a treatment for a type of tuberculosis (TB). The Gerson therapy was later used to treat other conditions, including cancer.

What Is The Theory Behind The Claim That The Gerson Therapy Is Useful In Treating Cancer?

The Gerson therapy is based on the idea that cancer develops when there are changes in cell metabolism because of the buildup of toxic substances in the body. Dr. Gerson said the disease process makes more toxins and the liver becomes overworked. According to Dr. Gerson, people with cancer also have too much sodium and too little potassium in the cells in their bodies, which causes tissue damage and weakened organs.

The goal of the Gerson therapy is to restore the body to health by repairing the liver and returning the metabolism to its normal state. According to Dr. Gerson, this can be done by removing toxins from the body and building up the immune system with diet and supplements. The enemas are said to widen the bile ducts of the liver so toxins can be released. According to Dr. Gerson, the liver is further overworked as the treatment regimen breaks down cancer cells and rids the body of toxins. Pancreatic enzymes are given to decrease the demands on the weakened liver and pancreas to make enzymes for digestion. An organic diet and nutritional supplements are used to boost the immune system and support the body as the regimen cleans the body of toxins. Foods low in sodium and high in potassium are said to help correct the tissue damage caused by having too much sodium in the cells.

How Is The Gerson Therapy Administered?

The Gerson therapy requires that the many details of its treatment plan be followed exactly. Some key parts of the regimen include the following:

- Drinking 13 glasses of juice a day. The juice must be freshly made from organic fruits and vegetables and be taken once every hour.
- Eating vegetarian meals of organically grown fruits, vegetables, and whole grains.
- Taking a number of supplements, including:
    - Potassium.
    - Lugol's Solution (potassium iodide, iodine, and water).
    - Coenzyme Q10 injected with vitamin B12. (The original regimen used crude liver extract instead of coenzyme Q10.)
    - Vitamins A, C, and B3 (niacin).
    - Flaxseed oil.
    - Pancreatic enzymes.
    - Pepsin (a stomach enzyme).
- Taking coffee or chamomile enemas regularly to remove toxins from the body.
- Preparing food without salt, spices, or oils, and without using aluminum cookware or utensils.

Have Any Preclinical (Laboratory Or Animal) Studies Been Conducted Using The Gerson Therapy?

No results of laboratory or animal studies have been published in scientific journals.

Have Any Side Effects Or Risks Been Reported From Use Of The Gerson Therapy?

Reports of three deaths that may be related to coffee enemas have been published. Taking too many enemas of any kind can cause changes in normal blood chemistry, chemicals that occur naturally in the body and keep the muscles, heart, and other organs working properly.

Is The Gerson Therapy Approved By The U.S. Food And Drug Administration (FDA) For Use As A Cancer Treatment In The United States?

The Gerson therapy has not been approved by the FDA for use as a treatment for cancer or any other disease.

Points To Consider

- The regimen is intended to "detoxify" the body while building up the immune system and raising the level of potassium in cells.
- No results of laboratory or animal studies are reported in the scientific literature contained in the Medical Literature Analysis and Retrieval System Online database.
- Few clinical studies of the Gerson therapy are found in the medical literature.

(Source: "Gerson Therapy (PDQ®)—Health Professional Version," National Cancer Institute (NCI).)

Part Six
Energy Medicine

Chapter 49

Acupuncture

What Is Acupuncture?

Acupuncture is a technique in which practitioners stimulate specific points on the body—most often by inserting thin needles through the skin. It is one of the practices used in traditional Chinese medicine (TCM).

Background

Acupuncture is part of TCM. TCM is a medical system that has been used for thousands of years to prevent, diagnose, and treat disease. Acupuncture is based on the belief that qi (vital energy) flows through the body along a network of paths, called meridians. Qi is said to affect a person's spiritual, emotional, mental, and physical condition.

How Is Acupuncture Administered?

The acupuncture method most well-known uses needles. Disposable, stainless steel needles that are slightly thicker than a human hair are inserted into the skin at acupoints. The acupuncture practitioner determines the correct acupoints to use for the problem being treated. The inserted needles may be twirled, moved up and down at different speeds and depths, heated, or charged with a weak electric current. There are other acupuncture methods that do not use needles.

(Source: "Acupuncture (PDQ®)–Patient Version," National Cancer Institute (NCI).)

About This Chapter: Text beginning with the heading "What Is Acupuncture?" is excerpted from "Acupuncture: In Depth," National Center for Complementary and Integrative Health (NCCIH), January 2016; Text under the heading "Acupuncture May Be Helpful For Chronic Pain: A Meta-Analysis" is excerpted from "Acupuncture May Be Helpful For Chronic Pain: A Meta-Analysis," National Center for Complementary and Integrative Health (NCCIH), September 10, 2012. Reviewed January 2018.

What The Science Says About The Effectiveness Of Acupuncture

Results from a number of studies suggest that acupuncture may help ease types of pain that are often chronic such as low-back pain, neck pain, and osteoarthritis/knee pain. It also may help reduce the frequency of tension headaches and prevent migraine headaches. Therefore, acupuncture appears to be a reasonable option for people with chronic pain to consider. However, clinical practice guidelines are inconsistent in recommendations about acupuncture.

The effects of acupuncture on the brain and body and how best to measure them are only beginning to be understood. Evidence suggests that many factors—like expectation and belief—that are unrelated to acupuncture needling may play important roles in the beneficial effects of acupuncture on pain.

For Low-Back Pain

- An analysis of data on participants in acupuncture studies looked at back and neck pain together and found that actual acupuncture was more helpful than either no acupuncture or simulated acupuncture.
- A review by the Agency for Healthcare Research and Quality (AHRQ) found that acupuncture relieved low-back pain immediately after treatment but not over longer periods of time.
- A systematic review of studies on acupuncture for low-back pain found strong evidence that combining acupuncture with usual care helps more than usual care alone. The same review also found strong evidence that there is no difference between the effects of actual and simulated acupuncture in people with low-back pain.
- Clinical practice guidelines issued by the American Pain Society (APS) and the American College of Physicians (ACP) recommends acupuncture as one of several nondrug approaches physicians should consider when patients with chronic low-back pain do not respond to self-care (practices that people can do by themselves, such as remaining active, applying heat, and taking pain-relieving medications).

For Neck Pain

- An analysis found that actual acupuncture was more helpful for neck pain than simulated acupuncture, but the analysis was based on a small amount of evidence (only three studies with small study populations).

- A large German study with more than 14,000 participants evaluated adding acupuncture to usual care for neck pain. The researchers found that participants reported greater pain relief than those who didn't receive it; the researchers didn't test actual acupuncture against simulated acupuncture.

For Osteoarthritis/Knee Pain

- An Australian clinical study involving 282 men and women showed that needle and laser acupuncture were modestly better at relieving knee pain from osteoarthritis than no treatment, but not better than simulated (sham) laser acupuncture. Participants received 8–12 actual and simulated acupuncture treatments over 12 weeks. These results are generally consistent with previous studies, which showed that acupuncture is consistently better than no treatment but not necessarily better than simulated acupuncture at relieving osteoarthritis pain.
- A major analysis of data on participants in acupuncture studies found that actual acupuncture was more helpful for osteoarthritis pain than simulated acupuncture or no acupuncture.
- A systematic review of studies of acupuncture for knee or hip osteoarthritis concluded that actual acupuncture was more helpful for osteoarthritis pain than either simulated acupuncture or no acupuncture. However, the difference between actual and simulated acupuncture was very small, while the difference between acupuncture and no acupuncture was large.

For Headache

- An analysis of data on individual participants in acupuncture studies looked at migraine and tension headaches. The analysis showed that actual acupuncture was more effective than either no acupuncture or simulated acupuncture in reducing headache frequency or severity.
- A systematic review of studies concluded that actual acupuncture, compared with simulated acupuncture or pain-relieving drugs, helped people with tension-type headaches. It suggested that actual acupuncture has a very slight advantage over simulated acupuncture in reducing tension-type headache intensity and the number of headache days per month.
- A systematic review found that adding acupuncture to basic care for migraines helped to reduce migraine frequency. However, in studies that compared actual acupuncture with

simulated acupuncture, researchers found that the differences between the two treatments may have been due to chance.

For Other Conditions

- Results of a systematic review that combined data from 11 clinical trials with more than 1,200 participants suggested that acupuncture (and acupuncture point stimulation) may help with certain symptoms associated with cancer treatments.
- There is not enough evidence to determine if acupuncture can help people with depression.
- Acupuncture has been promoted as a smoking cessation treatment since the 1970s, but research has not shown that it helps people quit the habit.

What Is Simulated Acupuncture?

In some clinical trials, researchers test a product or practice against an inactive product or technique (called a placebo) to see if the response is due to the test protocol or to something else. Many acupuncture trials rely on a technique called simulated acupuncture, which may use blunt-tipped retractable needles that touch the skin but do not penetrate (in real acupuncture, needles penetrate the skin). Researchers also may simulate acupuncture in other ways. However, in some instances, researchers have observed that simulated acupuncture resulted in some degree of pain relief.

What The Science Says About Safety And Side Effects Of Acupuncture

- Relatively few complications from using acupuncture have been reported. Still, complications have resulted from use of nonsterile needles and improper delivery of treatments.
- When not delivered properly, acupuncture can cause serious adverse effects, including infections, punctured organs, collapsed lungs, and injury to the central nervous system.
- The U.S. Food and Drug Administration (FDA) regulates acupuncture needles as medical devices for use by licensed practitioners and requires that needles be manufactured and labeled according to certain standards. For example, the FDA requires

that needles be sterile, nontoxic, and labeled for single use by qualified practitioners only.

Acupuncture May Be Helpful For Chronic Pain: A Meta-Analysis

A National Center for Complementary and Integrative Health (NCCIH)-funded study, employing individual patient data meta-analyses and published in the *Archives of Internal Medicine*, provides the most rigorous evidence to date that acupuncture may be helpful for chronic pain. In addition, results from the study provide robust evidence that the effects of acupuncture on pain are attributable to two components. The larger component includes factors such as the patient's belief that treatment will be effective, as well as placebo and other context effects. A smaller acupuncture-specific component involves such issues as the locations of specific needling points or depth of needling.

Although millions of Americans use acupuncture each year, often for chronic pain, there has been considerable controversy surrounding its value as a therapy and whether it is anything more than an elaborate placebo. Research exploring a number of possible mechanisms for acupuncture's pain-relieving effects is ongoing.

Researchers from the Acupuncture Trialists' Collaboration, a group that was established to synthesize data from high-quality randomized trials on acupuncture for chronic pain, conducted an analysis of individual patient data from 29 high-quality randomized controlled trials, including a total of 17,922 people. These trials investigated the use of acupuncture for back and neck pain, osteoarthritis, shoulder pain, or chronic headache.

For all pain types studied, the researchers found modest but statistically significant differences between acupuncture versus simulated acupuncture approaches (i.e., specific effects), and larger differences between acupuncture versus a no-acupuncture controls (i.e., nonspecific effects). (In traditional acupuncture, needles are inserted at specific points on the body. Simulated acupuncture includes a variety of approaches which mimic this procedure; some approaches do not pierce the skin or use specific points on the body.) The sizes of the effects were generally similar across all pain conditions studied.

The authors noted that these findings suggest that the total effects of acupuncture, as experienced by patients in clinical practice, are clinically relevant. They also noted that their study provides the most robust evidence to date that acupuncture is more than just placebo and a reasonable referral option for patients with chronic pain.

If You Want To Try Acupuncture

- Talk to your healthcare provider about it, especially if you're pregnant or nursing, or are thinking of using acupuncture to treat a child.
- Find an acupuncturist who's experienced working with your problem.
- Check credentials. Most states require a license to practice acupuncture.
- Don't use acupuncture as a replacement for conventional care.
- Don't rely on a diagnosis of disease by an acupuncturist who doesn't have conventional medical training.
- To help ensure coordinated and safe care, tell your healthcare providers about any complementary and alternative practices you use.

(Source: "Understanding Acupuncture," NIH News in Health, *National Institutes of Health (NIH).)*

Chapter 50

Magnet Therapy

Magnets have not been proven to work for any health-related purpose, yet static, or permanent, magnets are widely marketed for pain control.

About Magnets

A magnet produces a measurable force called a magnetic field. Static magnets have magnetic fields that do not change (unlike electromagnets, which generate magnetic fields only when electrical current flows through them). Magnets are usually made from metals (such as iron) or alloys (mixtures of metals, or of a metal and a nonmetal).

Magnets come in different strengths, often measured in units called gauss (G) or, alternatively, units called tesla (T; 1T=10,000 G). Magnets marketed for pain relief usually claim strengths of 300–5,000 G—many times stronger than the Earth's magnetic field (about 0.5 G) but much weaker than the magnets used for magnetic resonance imaging (MRI) machines (approximately 15,000 G or higher).

Magnets are often marketed for many different types of pain, including foot pain and back pain from conditions such as arthritis and fibromyalgia. Various products with magnets in them include shoe insoles, bracelets and other jewellery, mattress pads, and bandages.

About This Chapter: This chapter includes text excerpted from "Magnets," National Center for Complementary and Integrative Health (NCCIH), February 2013. Reviewed January 2018.

Different types of magnets have been studied for pain.

- **Static or permanent magnets.** Static magnets have magnetic fields that do not change. The activity of electrons in the metal causes it to be magnetic. These magnets usually aren't very strong and are often put in products such as shoe insoles, headbands, bracelets, and more.
- **Electromagnets.** This type of magnet is created when electrical current charges the metal, making it magnetic. Devices with electromagnets in them are also marketed for health purposes.

(Source: "Magnets For Pain," National Center for Complementary and Integrative Health (NCCIH).)

Safety And Side Effects

- Magnets may not be safe for some people, such as those who use a pacemaker or an insulin pump; magnets may interfere with the functioning of the medical device. Otherwise, magnets are generally considered safe when applied to the skin.
- Reports of side effects or complications have been rare.

- Beyond interference with medical devices, there isn't much good information on the possible side effects of magnets, but few problems have been reported.
- Children may swallow or accidentally inhale small magnets, which can be deadly.
- Do not use static magnets or electromagnets that you can buy without a prescription to postpone seeing a healthcare provider about pain or any other medical problem.

(Source: "Magnets For Pain," National Center for Complementary and Integrative Health (NCCIH).)

What The Science Says About Magnets For Pain

Scientific evidence does not support the use of magnets for pain relief. Preliminary studies looking at different types of pain—such as knee, hip, wrist, foot, back, and pelvic pain—have had mixed results. Some of these studies, including a clinical trial sponsored by the National Institutes of Health (NIH) that looked at back pain in a small group of people, have suggested a benefit from using magnets.

However, many studies have not been of high quality; they included a small number of participants, were too short, and/or were inadequately controlled. The majority of rigorous trials have found no effect on pain.

If You Are Considering Using Magnets

- Do not use magnets or any unproven health practice to replace conventional healthcare or to postpone seeing a healthcare provider about pain or any other medical problem.
- Tell all your healthcare providers about any complementary or integrative health approaches you use. Give them a full picture of what you do to manage your health. This will help ensure coordinated and safe care.

Chapter 51

Therapeutic Touch

What Is Therapeutic Touch?

Therapeutic touch, sometimes called "laying on of hands," is a type of therapy that practitioners say promotes relaxation, pain relief, healing, and the restoration of balanced energy fields. Although it is based on ancient principles, modern therapeutic touch was developed in the 1970s by Dolores Krieger, a professor of nursing, and Dora Kunz, a natural healer and a theosophy.. And although the effectiveness of therapeutic touch remains controversial, their methods have since been taught to many thousands of people, including health professionals and lay practitioners.

> **Therapeutic Touch: Definition**
>
> A form of complementary and alternative medicine based on the belief that vital energy flows through the human body. This energy is said to be balanced or made stronger by practitioners who pass their hands over, or gently touch, a patient's body. Therapeutic touch is a type of energy therapy. Also called healing touch (HT).
>
> *(Source: "NCI Dictionary Of Cancer Terms," National Cancer Institute (NCI).)*

Despite the name, practitioners of therapeutic touch generally place their hands two to four inches over an individual's body, passing them from head to toe in order to identify energy that is out of balance. By doing so, the practitioner interacts with the individual's energy field and can consciously direct or modulate the person's energies. According to proponents, mind, body, and emotions are components of a complex energy field. The therapy works on the principle that when these three (mind, body, and emotions) are balanced they are an indication of good health, whereas when there is an imbalance the result is bad health.

Energy Field

In the ancient health systems of such civilizations as India and China, an energy field is known as life energy. It is present throughout the body and is responsible for the maintenance of psychological, physiological, and spiritual functions. In the Indian ayurvedic system, it is called "prana," and in traditional Chinese medicine, it is "qi." In these and many other cultures, correcting disruptions or imbalances in the life energy is a key part of healthcare.

How Is Therapeutic Touch Performed?

A typical session of therapeutic touch will last for approximately 15–30 minutes, during which the individual will sit in a chair or lie down, fully clothed. The session starts with the practitioner asking the client about his or her healing goals and the problems being faced. Then the practitioner uses sweeping hand motions above the individual to identify and attempt to balance the energy field in and around the body. The following are some of the steps that may be followed by the practitioner during a therapeutic touch session:

- **Centering.** The practitioner focuses to a level of calm.
- **Assessment.** The client's energy field is appraised.
- **Intervention.** If an imbalance is identified, the practitioner clears and mobilizes the individual's energy field and redirects energy to achieve wholeness and balance in the field.
- **Evaluation and closure.** The practitioner evaluates the effectiveness of the treatment. If the individual has any questions, the practitioner answers them and asks for feedback.

Benefits Of Therapeutic Touch

Therapeutic touch aims to help an individual discover his or her own healing process and restore wholeness at physical, mental, and emotional levels. The two most reliable and immediate effects of therapeutic touch are said to be pain relief and relaxation. The therapy helps stimulating the body's natural healing but does not necessarily claim to cure any illness.

Some of the benefits of therapeutic touch, as described by practitioners and clients, are discussed below.

- Therapeutic touch is said to be effective on people of all ages.
- Therapeutic touch stimulates cell growth.
- The process can relieve tension headaches and reduce pain, including that stemming from burns, osteoarthritis, or surgery.
- It helps improve joint function in people affected by arthritis.
- It can reduce stress in patients with cancer and heart disease.
- Some research suggests that the therapy helps reduce cholesterol levels, improve breathing, and lower blood pressure.
- Therapeutic touch can ease difficult pregnancies.
- Along with conventional medical treatment, the therapy can help patients with such other conditions as lupus, chronic pain, Alzheimer disease, addictions, allergies, sleep apnea, fibromyalgia, bronchitis, and restless legs syndrome.
- Some people experience significant emotional and spiritual change after the therapy. They may gain more self-confidence and self-control.

Healing Touch (HT) For Cancer Treatment

Healing touch (HT) is a complementary and alternative medicines (CAM) treatment frequently used by cancer patients to reduce adverse side effects of chemotherapy and radiation and to enhance immunity. HT is classified by National Institutes of Health (NIH) as a "biofield" therapy as its effects are proposed to be secondary to manipulation of "energy fields" around the body of a patient. A recent meta-analysis has demonstrated relatively large effects of HT on well-being and on physiological parameters, even from brief treatments.

(Source: "Healing Touch, Quality Of Life, And Immunity During Breast Cancer Treatment," ClinicalTrials.gov, National Institutes of Health (NIH).)

Risks Of Therapeutic Touch

Since therapeutic touch is noninvasive and is not generally used as a major form of treatment for any serious health conditions, it comes with very few risks. After a therapeutic touch session, the individual can feel lightheaded, thirsty, and may need to urinate. In most cases, the light-headedness may last for around 15 minutes, and the individual can feel thirsty for a few days. However, some therapeutic practitioners say the therapy can cause mild fever and some inflammation, and some have found that too much energy can cause increased pain and leave the individual frustrated, anxious, and restless. Practitioners also suggest that therapeutic touch should not be done in areas of the body affected with cancer.

If an individual has been abused physically or sexually in the past, it is best discussed with the practitioner before the session begins, even though the therapy does not involve touching. Children, the elderly, and extremely sick people should be treated only for a short period of time, according to some therapeutic practitioners.

References

1. "Therapeutic Touch," University of Maryland Medical Center, February 4, 2016.
2. "Therapeutic Touch," University of Minnesota, October 29, 2008.
3. "Therapeutic Touch: Topic Overview," WebMD, December 22, 2007.
4. "Understanding Therapeutic Touch," Therapeutic Touch Network of Ontario, September 1, 2007.

Chapter 52

Reiki

What Is Reiki?

Reiki is a complementary health approach in which practitioners place their hands lightly on or just above a person, with the goal of facilitating the person's own healing response.

- Reiki is based on an Eastern belief in an energy that supports the body's innate or natural healing abilities. However, there isn't any scientific evidence that such an energy exists.
- Reiki has been studied for a variety of conditions, including pain, anxiety, fatigue, and depression.

What The Anecdotal Literature Says About Reiki For Treating Fibromyalgia

Fibromyalgia is a common, chronic condition that causes muscle pain and fatigue. People with fibromyalgia often turn to complementary health approaches, such as Reiki, to help relieve their pain. Reiki is a form of energy medicine in which the practitioner seeks to transmit a "universal healing energy" to a person, either from a distance or through light touch. In general, evidence for energy medicine is scant, but anecdotal (subjective) literature suggests that Reiki can improve pain control and psychological well-being with few or no adverse effects.

(Source: "Reiki Does Not Improve Fibromyalgia Symptoms In Clinical Trial," National Center for Complementary and Integrative Health (NCCIH).)

About This Chapter: This chapter includes text excerpted from "Reiki: In Depth," National Center for Complementary and Integrative Health (NCCIH), October 2015.

What The Science Says About The Effectiveness Of Reiki

Several groups of experts have evaluated the evidence on Reiki, and all of them have concluded that it's uncertain whether Reiki is helpful.

Only a small number of studies of Reiki have been completed, and most of them included only a few people. Different studies looked at different health conditions making it hard to compare their results. Many of the studies didn't compare Reiki with both sham (simulated) Reiki and with no treatment. Studies that include both of these comparisons are usually the most informative.

What The Science Says About The Safety Of Reiki

Reiki appears to be generally safe. In studies of Reiki, side effects were no more common among participants who received Reiki than among those who didn't receive it.

More To Consider

- Reiki should not be used to replace conventional care or to postpone seeing a healthcare provider about a health problem. If you have severe or long-lasting symptoms, see your healthcare provider. You may have a health problem that needs prompt treatment.
- Tell all your healthcare providers about any complementary health approaches you use. Give them a full picture of what you do to manage your health. This will help ensure coordinated and safe care.

Part Seven
Creative Arts Therapies

Chapter 53

Art Therapies

What Is Art Therapy?

Art therapy is based on the idea that the creative process of art making is healing and life enhancing, and is a form of nonverbal communication of thoughts and feelings. Art therapy encourages personal growth, increases self-understanding and assists in emotional reparation. Participation in this treatment modality does not require any artistic training. The therapists involved in providing this treatment are all trained registered/licensed art therapists.

Art therapy helps individuals to:

- Create meaning;
- Achieve insight;
- Find relief from overwhelming emotions or trauma and posttraumatic stress disorder (PTSD);
- Resolve conflicts and problems, enrich daily life;
- Achieve an increased sense of well-being.

About This Chapter: Text under the heading "What Is Art Therapy?" is excerpted from "VA Palo Alto Health Care System—What Is Art Therapy?" U.S. Department of Veterans Affairs (VA), April 11, 2017; Text under the heading "Creative Art Therapy And The Integrated Healthcare Model" is excerpted from "Creative Arts Therapy A Useful Tool For Military Patients," National Endowment For The Arts (NEA), November 12, 2015; Text under the heading "Historical Context Of Research Into The Arts And Health" is excerpted from "The National Endowment For The Arts Guide To Community-Engaged Research In The Arts And Health," National Endowment For The Arts (NEA), December 2016; Text under the heading "How Arts Can Aid Trauma Recovery" is excerpted from "Calm Through Creativity: How Arts Can Aid Trauma Recovery," Family and Youth Services Bureau (FYSB), December 18, 2013. Reviewed January 2018; Text under the heading "Creative Art Therapists" is excerpted from "You're A What? Art Therapist," U.S. Bureau of Labor Statistics (BLS), U.S. Department of Labor (DOL), April 2015.

Creative Art Therapy And The Integrated Healthcare Model

Creative arts therapy is a noninvasive and cost-effective medical treatment in which certified creative arts therapists work closely with other health professionals to create individual treatment plans with measurable outcomes. Patients may receive therapies such as painting, ceramics, music therapy, and therapeutic writing to improve health conditions for a wide range of medical, physical, neurological, and psychological health issues, such as depression, anxiety, cognitive function, memory, and impaired motor skills. Patients have described how art therapy activities have improved their cognitive skills and ability to process trauma and confront issues relating to frustrations, transitions, and grief.

Historical Context Of Research Into The Arts And Health

Therapeutic uses of the arts have been documented since antiquity. For centuries, artists, philosophers, physicians, and others have proposed specific benefits of the arts for health and well-being. For instance, early examples about the therapeutic value of music date back at least to the 18th century, when references to music appeared in medical texts and references to medicine in music treatises. An interest in using the arts to influence health developed substantially in the 20th century when arts professionals formalized distinct arts therapies by founding professional organizations and creating educational training programs. Among these interventions are music therapy, visual art therapy, dance/movement therapy, drama therapy, and several other genre-based forms of creative arts therapy.

How Arts Can Aid Trauma Recovery

It takes a lot of effort for the brain to deal with trauma. Whether because of post-traumatic stress disorder or the many adaptive behaviors that victims use instinctively in threatening situations, the traumatized brain is constantly on high-alert, particularly its lower regions, where survival instincts originate. Simple artistic activities like drawing or sculpting clay can soothe those lower regions, which is why arts therapists argue that their methods can help trauma victims calm down and release some of that mental tension. These evidence-informed therapies use creativity to raise victims' awareness of their physical and mental states and build resilience and a sense of safety. Counselor and author Cathy Malchiodi, who has pioneered trauma-informed art therapy and trauma-informed expressive arts therapy, claims that the use of music, art and other creative activities grant victims a means of expressing the effects of trauma even after therapy ends.

When the lower-brain's instincts are over-activated, they can inhibit people's ability to perform higher cognitive functions until they have started healing from trauma. "Teens who are stressed may have difficulty answering questions about their drug use, or about making goals and plans for the future," Malchiodi says. However, as she and other researchers have found, these effects can be reversed with therapies that rebuild the brain from the ground up.

Nancy Gerber, Director of the PhD Program in Creative Arts Therapies at Drexel University, explains that expressive arts support trauma recovery, especially for those victims who were traumatized or seek treatment at a young age, because they engage the regions of the brain that develop earlier in life. "A lot of kids in adolescence struggle with language," she says. "They know how to talk but they don't always know how to talk with emotional intelligence. The idea [of arts therapy] is that images are a form of cognition, a way of knowing. They develop very early in our lives: little kids point at things before they have a word for them. These images provide a history for the early life, and when we grow up we don't have a word for that." Simply put, arts therapy helps trauma victims reconnect with that image-based part of the brain, a process which calms the parts of the brain that have been overworked by trauma.

Here's how it works:

Step 1: Getting in touch with the "lower brain"

Traumatic stress manifests differently for different people; victims may be withdrawn and uncommunicative, or wild and confrontational. (In therapeutic terms, this is referred to as "internalizing" or "externalizing" one's feelings.) In her previous work at an inpatient psychiatric hospital, mostly focused on adolescents, Gerber included drawing in every young patient's intake process. She would then share the drawings with staff when they met to decide on a treatment plan. It was particularly useful for those young people who couldn't easily express their experiences verbally.

"The art provides a different dimension that most of us don't know how to say," Gerber says. "A picture can tell a story about our internal life that isn't accessible in words."

Malchiodi begins her therapy by observing her clients to infer what kind of activities would help them best. Some may benefit from therapies that help them loosen up, such as movement activities with music. Others need to do something that will help calm them down and focus, such as drawing or painting.

In one treatment, she gives individuals a rubber duck and asks them to build a safe place for it using feathers, paper plates, leaves, fabric and other materials.

"This highly sensory experience, where you can actually feel the nest, pond, or whatever you build, engages the lower parts of your brain, whereas simply drawing a safe place or depicting goals require higher cognitive areas," Malchiodi explains.

Step 2: Becoming more expressive

For young and older people alike, the experience of traumatic events can be difficult to express in words. So Malchiodi uses the first step to get them feeling calmer and more creatively expressive. Then she engages them in storytelling activities that use higher cognitive areas. For example, she might ask, "If you could draw a bridge that starts in the past and goes into the future, show me where you are on the bridge," or to depict one's family in any way they choose to depict it.

Gerber says that expressive arts therapy allows victims to deal with trauma in the same deeply emotional way that they experience it, which in turn prepares them to address it more fully. "They no longer had to act out," she says of her clients. "They could have conversations about how they saw themselves and the world."

Malchiodi saw similar results in her young people. "Trauma memories are sensory memories," she says, "meaning that people feel them in their bodies and react with their bodies." Creativity can help them make that leap to full understanding and expression.

Creative Art Therapists

What They Do

Art therapists work in different settings with different types of clients. Some are in schools, where they work with students of all ages and meet with them in groups or one-on-one. Many others work in medical settings, such as community clinics and psychiatric hospitals, where they may help people who have a physical or mental illness. Still others have their own practice, serving clients with various needs.

But no matter where they work or who their clients are, art therapists use art and psychology on the job.

Art. Every client has different needs, but for some, the process of creating may be valuable on its own. For example, people who have trouble focusing may become more grounded when working with clay. Using paints, in contrast, can help people release emotion.

Art therapists design projects using their understanding of how art media and techniques can influence people. For example, a therapist may ask students to create an image showing parts of their past that they would like to leave behind. Then, he or she may have them create an image that depicts their future and shows the positive elements they hope to build on. This helps them think about what they want to change about themselves, what they want to be.

Psychology. Knowledge of psychology allows an art therapist to help clients understand themselves and work toward specific goals. The art therapist engages clients in reflection about the art that they have created. It's all about exploring things they're trying to process that they can't verbally communicate. Sometimes they're not ready to talk, but just having a person there helps. When clients are ready to process their thoughts, the art therapist might discuss ways to help them deal with whatever they're facing. For example, an art therapist might work with clients to develop coping skills or strategies for changing behavior.

Chapter 54

Music Therapy

Music has been around since ancient times. It is part of every known culture. It can get your foot tapping, lift your mood, and even help you recall a distant memory. Did you know that music can bring other health benefits? Scientists are exploring the different ways music stimulates healthier bodies and minds.

"When you listen to or create music, it affects how you think, feel, move, and more," says neuroscientist Dr. Robert Finkelstein, who coleads National Institutes of Health's (NIH) music and health initiative.

"At present, modern technologies are helping researchers learn more about how the brain works, what parts of the brain respond to music, and how music might help ease symptoms of certain diseases and conditions," he explains.

The Power Of Music

Several well-controlled studies have found that listening to music can alleviate pain or reduce the need for pain medications. Other research suggests that music can benefit heart disease patients by reducing their blood pressure, heart rate, and anxiety. Music therapy has also been shown to lift the spirits of patients with depression. Making music yourself—either playing instruments or singing—can have therapeutic effects as well.

(Source: "Strike A Chord For Health—Music Matters For Body And Mind," NIH News in Health, *National Institutes of Health (NIH).)*

About This Chapter: This chapter includes text excerpted from "Sound Health—Music Gets You Moving And More," *NIH News in Health*, National Institutes of Health (NIH), January 2018.

Your Brain On Music

The brain is a complex processing hub. It's the control center of your nervous system, the network of nerve cells that carry messages to and from your body and the brain. A healthy brain tries to make sense of the world around you and the constant information it receives, including sound and music.

"Sound is an important and profound force in our lives," explains Northwestern University (NU) neuroscientist Dr. Nina Kraus. "The more we exercise our sound processing in the brain, the better the brain becomes at making sense of sound and the world around us. Music does this more than any other sound."

Music and other sounds enter the ear as sound waves. These create vibrations on our eardrum that are transformed into electrical signals. The electrical signals travel up the auditory nerve to the brain's auditory cortex. This brain area interprets the sound into something we recognize and understand.

"When you make music, it engages many different areas of the brain, including visual, auditory and motor areas," says neuroscientist Dr. Gottfried Schlaug of Harvard Medical School. "That's why music-making is also of potential interest in treating neurological disorders."

(Source: "Strike A Chord For Health—Music Matters For Body And Mind," NIH News in Health, *National Institutes of Health (NIH).)*

But music affects more than the brain areas that process sound. Using techniques that take pictures of the brain, like functional magnetic resonance imaging or functional MRI (fMRI), scientists have found that music affects other brain areas. When music stimulates the brain, it shows up on brain images as flickers of bright light. Studies have shown that music "lights up" brain areas involved in emotion, memory, and even physical movement.

"Music can help facilitate movement," Finkelstein explains. NIH-funded scientists are investigating whether music can help patients with movement disorders, like Parkinson disease (PD). Patients with this condition slowly lose their ability to walk and move over time.

"Studies show that when a certain beat is embedded in music, it can help people with PD walk," Finkelstein says. Another study is looking at how dance compares to other types of exercise in people with PD.

There's also evidence that music may be helpful for people with other health conditions, including Alzheimer disease (AD), dementia, traumatic brain injury (TBI), stroke, aphasia, autism, and hearing loss.

Building Strong Minds

Playing a musical instrument engages many parts of the brain at once. This can especially benefit children and teens, whose brains are still developing. Introducing music to young kids can positively influence their ability to focus, how they act, and language development.

Kraus's research team at Northwestern studies how musical training influences brain development. They found that music has positive effects on kids' learning abilities, even when the training starts as late as high school.

"The teens in our study showed biological changes in the brain after two years of participating in consistent music-making activities in school," she explains. Kraus says that these changes affect learning ability and can help improve skills like reading and writing. These benefits can be long lasting, too.

"Once you teach your brain how to respond to sound effectively it continues to do that well beyond when the music lessons stop," Kraus explains. "A little music goes a long way, but the longer you play, the stronger your brain becomes."

Being musical may also protect you from hearing loss as you age. We naturally lose our hearing ability over time. In particular, it becomes harder to hear conversations in a loud environment. But researchers have found that musicians are better at picking out a person's voice in a noisy background.

Music Therapy

Listening to and making music on your own can bring health benefits. But some people may also benefit from the help of a board-certified music therapist. Music therapists are trained in how to use music to meet the mental, social, and physical needs of people with different health conditions.

"Music therapy can take many forms that go beyond listening to music," explains Dr. Sheri Robb, a music therapist and behavioral intervention researcher at Indiana University.

Music therapists can use certain parts of music, like the rhythm or melody, to help people regain abilities they've lost from a brain injury or developmental disability. For example, a person who's had a stroke may be able to sing words, but not speak them.

Music therapists also rely on the social qualities of music. Shared musical experiences can help a family member connect with a loved one who has dementia. Music can also be used to help young people with behavior disorders learn ways to manage their emotions.

Robb's research focuses on developing and testing music therapy interventions for children and teens with cancer and their families. In one study, music therapists helped young people undergoing high-risk cancer treatments to write song lyrics and create music videos about what was most important to them.

"With the help of music therapists, these teenagers were able to identify their strengths and positive ways to cope, remain connected with family and friends, and improve communication during a challenging time," Robb explains.

Music In Your Life

Music can offer many health benefits, but it may not be helpful for everyone. Traumatic injuries and brain conditions can change the way a person perceives and responds to music. Some people may find some types of music overstimulating. Others may find that certain music brings up emotional or traumatic memories.

"It's important for healthcare providers to identify and understand when music isn't helpful and may be harmful," Robb says. "And this is an area where music therapists can be helpful."

As scientists continue to learn more about music and the brain, try striking a chord for your health. Whether you're looking to boost your mood, stay connected to others, or improve symptoms of a health condition, add a little music to your life.

"Think of music like physical fitness or what you eat," Kraus says. "To see the most health benefits, try to include music as a regular, consistent part of your life. It's never too late to add music to your life."

Ways To Add More Music To Your Life

- Listen to music during the day, like on your way to work or during exercise.
- Sing and dance while you're doing chores or cooking meals.
- Play a musical instrument. Consider taking lessons or joining friends to make music.
- Attend concerts, plays, and other community music activities in your area.
- Encourage your kids to listen to music, sing, play an instrument, or participate in music programs at school.

- Ask your doctor if music therapy is right for you. Consider working with a board-certified music therapist to improve your health.

There is some evidence that music therapy may help to improve some social and behavioral skills in children with ASD. A 2014 review of scientific studies concluded that music therapy may help children with ASD to improve their skills in areas such as social interaction and communication, and may also contribute to increasing social adaptation skills.

(Source: "7 Things To Know About Complementary Health Approaches For ASD," National Center for Complementary and Integrative Health (NCCIH).)

Part Eight

CAM Treatments For Cancer And Other Diseases And Conditions

Chapter 55

Cancer And Complementary Health Therapies

People with cancer want to do everything they can to combat the disease, manage its symptoms, and cope with the side effects of treatment. Many turn to complementary health approaches, including natural products, such as herbs (botanicals) and other dietary supplements, and mind and body practices, such as acupuncture, massage, and yoga.

This chapter provides an introductory overview of complementary health approaches that have been studied for cancer prevention, treatment of the disease, or symptom management, including what the science says about their effectiveness and any concerns that have been raised about their safety.

About Cancer

Cancer is a term for diseases in which abnormal cells divide without control. Cancer cells can invade nearby tissues and spread to other parts of the body through the bloodstream and the lymph system. Although cancer is the second leading cause of death in the United States, improvements in screening, detection, treatment, and care have increased the number of cancer survivors, and experts expect the number of survivors to continue to increase in the coming years.

About Complementary Health Approaches

Complementary health approaches are a group of diverse medical and healthcare systems, practices, and products whose origins come from outside of mainstream medicine. They

About This Chapter: This chapter includes text excerpted from "Cancer: In Depth," National Center for Complementary and Integrative Health (NCCIH), July 2014. Reviewed January 2018.

include such products and practices as herbal supplements, other dietary supplements, meditation, spinal manipulation, and acupuncture.

The same careful scientific evaluation that is used to assess conventional therapies should be used to evaluate complementary approaches. Some complementary approaches are beginning to find a place in cancer treatment—not as cures, but as additions to treatment plans that may help patients cope with disease symptoms and side effects of treatment and improve their quality of life.

Use Of Complementary Health Approaches For Cancer

Many people who've been diagnosed with cancer use complementary health approaches.

- According to National Health Interview Survey (NHIS), which included a comprehensive survey on the use of complementary health approaches by Americans, 65 percent of respondents who had ever been diagnosed with cancer had used complementary approaches, as compared to 53 percent of other respondents. Those who had been diagnosed with cancer were more likely than others to have used complementary approaches for general wellness, immune enhancement, and pain management.
- Other surveys have also found that use of complementary health approaches is common among people who've been diagnosed with cancer, although estimates of use vary widely. Some data indicate that the likelihood of using complementary approaches varies with the type of cancer and with factors such as sex, age, and ethnicity. The results of surveys from 18 countries show that use of complementary approaches by people who had been diagnosed with cancer was more common in North America than in Australia/New Zealand or Europe and that use had increased since the 1970s and especially since 2000.
- Surveys have also shown that many people with cancer don't tell their healthcare providers about their use of complementary health approaches. In the NHIS, survey respondents who had been diagnosed with cancer told their healthcare providers about 15 percent of their herb use and 23 percent of their total use of complementary approaches. In other studies, between 32 and 69 percent of cancer patients and survivors who used dietary supplements or other complementary approaches reported that they discussed these approaches with their physicians. The differences in the reported percentages may reflect differences in the definitions of complementary approaches used in the studies, as well as differences in the communication practices of different groups of patients.

What The Science Says About The Safety And Side Effects Of Complementary Health Approaches For Cancer

- Delaying conventional cancer treatment can decrease the chances of remission or cure. Don't use unproven products or practices to postpone or replace conventional medical treatment for cancer.
- Some complementary health approaches may interfere with cancer treatments or be unsafe for cancer patients. For example, the herb St. John's wort, which is sometimes used for depression, can make some cancer drugs less effective.
- Other complementary approaches may be harmful if used inappropriately. For example, to make massage therapy safe for people with cancer, it may be necessary to avoid massaging places on the body that are directly affected by the disease or its treatment (for example, areas where the skin is sensitive following radiation therapy).
- People who've been diagnosed with cancer should consult the healthcare providers who are treating them for cancer before using any complementary health approach for any purpose—whether or not it's cancer-related.

What The Science Says About The Effectiveness Of Complementary Health Approaches For Cancer

No complementary health product or practice has been proven to cure cancer. Some complementary approaches may help people manage cancer symptoms or treatment side effects and improve their quality of life.

Incorporating Complementary Health Approaches Into Cancer Care

The Society for Integrative Oncology (SIO) issued evidence-based clinical practice guidelines for healthcare providers to consider when incorporating complementary health approaches in the care of cancer patients. The guidelines point out that, when used in addition to conventional therapies, some of these approaches help to control symptoms and enhance patients' well-being. The guidelines warn, however, that unproven methods shouldn't be used in place of conventional treatment because delayed treatment of cancer reduces the likelihood of a remission or cure.

The following sections provide an overview of the research status of some commonly used complementary approaches, highlighting results from a few reviews and studies focusing on preventing and treating the disease, as well as managing cancer symptoms and treatment side effects.

Complementary Health Approaches For Cancer Symptoms And Treatment Side Effects

Some complementary health approaches, such as acupuncture, massage therapy, mindfulness-based stress reduction, and yoga, may help people manage cancer symptoms or the side effects of treatment. However, some approaches may interfere with conventional cancer treatment or have other risks. People who have been diagnosed with cancer should consult their healthcare providers before using any complementary health approach.

- There is substantial evidence that acupuncture can help to manage treatment-related nausea and vomiting in cancer patients. There isn't enough evidence to judge whether acupuncture relieves cancer pain or other symptoms such as treatment-related hot flashes. Complications from acupuncture are rare, as long as the acupuncturist uses sterile needles and proper procedures. Chemotherapy and radiation therapy weaken the body's immune system, so it's especially important for acupuncturists to follow strict clean-needle procedures when treating cancer patients.
- Recent studies suggest that the herb ginger may help to control nausea related to cancer chemotherapy when used in addition to conventional antinausea medication.
- Studies suggest that massage therapy may help to relieve symptoms experienced by people with cancer, such as pain, nausea, anxiety, and depression. However, investigators haven't reached any conclusions about the effects of massage therapy because of the limited amount of rigorous research in this field. People with cancer should consult their healthcare providers before having massage therapy to find out if any special precautions are needed. The massage therapist shouldn't use deep or intense pressure without the healthcare providers approval and may need to avoid certain sites, such as areas directly over a tumor or those where the skin is sensitive following radiation therapy.
- There is evidence that mindfulness-based stress reduction, a type of meditation training, can help cancer patients relieve anxiety, stress, fatigue, and general mood and sleep disturbances, thus improving their quality of life. Most participants in mindfulness studies have been patients with early-stage cancer, primarily breast cancer, so the evidence favoring mindfulness training is strongest for this group of patients.

- Preliminary evidence indicates that yoga may help to improve anxiety, depression, distress, and stress in people with cancer. It also may help to lessen fatigue in breast cancer patients and survivors. However, only a small number of yoga studies in cancer patients have been completed, and some of the research hasn't been of the highest quality. Because yoga involves physical activities, it's important for people with cancer to talk with their healthcare providers in advance to find out whether any aspects of yoga might be unsafe for them.
- Various studies suggest possible benefits of hypnosis, relaxation therapies, and biofeedback to help patients manage cancer symptoms and treatment side effects.
- A review of the research literature on herbal supplements and cancer concluded that although several herbs have shown promise for managing side effects and symptoms such as nausea and vomiting, pain, fatigue, and insomnia, the scientific evidence is limited, and many clinical trials haven't been well designed. Use of herbs for managing symptoms also raises concerns about potential negative interactions with conventional cancer treatments.

Complementary Health Approaches For Cancer Treatment

This section discusses complementary health approaches to directly treat cancer (that is, to try to cure the disease or cause a remission).

No complementary approach has cured cancer or caused it to go into remission. Some products or practices that have been advocated for cancer treatment may interfere with conventional cancer treatments or have other risks. People who've been diagnosed with cancer should consult their healthcare providers before using any complementary health approach.

- Studies on whether herbal supplements or substances derived from them might be of value in cancer treatment are in their early stages, and scientific evidence is limited. Herbal supplements may have side effects, and some may interact in harmful ways with drugs, including drugs used in cancer treatment.
- The effects of taking vitamin and mineral supplements, including antioxidant supplements, during cancer treatment are uncertain. National Cancer Institute (NCI) advises cancer patients to talk to their healthcare providers before taking any supplements.
- A National Center for Complementary and Integrative Health (NCCIH)-supported trial of a standardized shark cartilage extract, taken in addition to chemotherapy and radiation therapy, showed no benefit in patients with advanced lung cancer. An earlier,

smaller study in patients with advanced breast or colorectal cancers also showed no benefit from the addition of shark cartilage to conventional treatment.

- A systematic review of research on laetrile found no evidence that it's effective as a cancer treatment. Laetrile can be toxic, especially if taken orally, because it contains cyanide.

Complementary Health Approaches For Cancer Prevention

A large clinical trial has shown that taking a multivitamin/mineral supplement may slightly reduce the risk of cancer in older men. No other complementary health approach has been shown to be helpful in preventing cancer, and some have been linked with increased health risks.

Other Natural Products. A systematic review of 51 studies with more than 1.6 million participants found "insufficient and conflicting" evidence regarding an association between consuming green tea and cancer prevention. Several other natural products, including *Ginkgo biloba*, isoflavones, noni, pomegranate, and grape seed extract, have been investigated for possible cancer-preventive effects, but the evidence on these substances is too limited for any conclusions to be reached.

Keep In Mind

- Unproven products or practices should not be used to replace or delay conventional medical treatment for cancer.
- Some complementary approaches can interfere with standard cancer treatments or have special risks for people who've been diagnosed with cancer. Before using any complementary health approach, people who've been diagnosed with cancer should talk with their healthcare providers to make sure that all aspects of their care work together.
- Tell all your healthcare providers about any complementary health approaches you use. Give them a full picture of what you do to manage your health. This will help ensure coordinated and safe care.

Chapter 56

CAM For Pain Management

What Is Chronic Pain And Why Is It Important?

Chronic pain is pain that lasts more than several months (variously defined as 3–6 months, but certainly longer than "normal healing"). It's a very common problem. Results from National Health Interview Survey (NHIS) show that individuals with severe pain had worse health, used more healthcare, and had more disability than those with less severe pain.

What The Science Says About Complementary Health Approaches For Chronic Pain

The scientific evidence suggests that some complementary health approaches may help people manage chronic pain.

This chapter highlights the research status of some approaches used for common kinds of pain.

Chronic Pain In General

Some research has looked at the effects of complementary approaches on chronic pain in general rather than on specific painful conditions.

- An evaluation of studies on active self-care complementary approaches (approaches that individuals can do themselves after being taught the technique) found that there is some evidence in favor of using yoga, tai chi, and music for self-management of chronic pain

---

About This Chapter: This chapter includes text excerpted from "Chronic Pain: In Depth," National Center for Complementary and Integrative Health (NCCIH), September 2016.

symptoms, but not enough to justify a strong recommendation for their use. The evidence is insufficient, according to this evaluation, to allow conclusions to be reached about other self-care approaches such as mindfulness/meditation, relaxation techniques, and qi gong.

- An evaluation of the research on mindfulness-based interventions found they may be helpful for patients with chronic pain, with effectiveness similar to that of cognitive-behavioral approaches.
- Research shows that hypnosis is moderately effective in managing chronic pain, when compared to usual medical care. However, the effectiveness of hypnosis can vary substantially from one person to another.
- There's some evidence that cannabinoids (substances from marijuana) might be helpful for chronic neuropathic or cancer pain.

Low-Back Pain

- A combined analysis of data from several studies concludes that acupuncture is a reasonable option to consider for chronic low-back pain. How acupuncture works to relieve pain is unclear. Current evidence suggests other factors—like expectation and belief—that are unrelated to acupuncture needling may play important roles in the beneficial effects of acupuncture on pain. A review of studies conducted in the United States found evidence that acupuncture can help some patients manage low-back pain.

Acupuncture therapy involves inserting very fine needles at a variety of points in the body, and has been shown to be effective in treating symptoms resulting from a wide range of conditions. It has long been known to activate endorphins, the body's natural pain relievers. Acupuncture may be effective for patients who suffer from:

- Pain associated with an injury or illness
- Nausea and vomiting after an operation
- Nausea and vomiting related to chemotherapy
- Knee pain from osteoarthritis
- Low back pain
- Depression or other mental health concerns
- Substance dependency

(Source: "Acupuncture Therapy For Veteran Pain," U.S. Department of Veterans Affairs (VA).)

- Massage might provide short-term relief from low-back pain, but the evidence is not of high quality. Massage has not been shown to have long-term benefits on low-back pain.
- There is some evidence that progressive relaxation may help relieve low-back pain, but studies on this topic have not been of the highest quality.
- Spinal manipulation appears to be as effective as other therapies commonly used for chronic low-back pain, such as physical therapy, exercise, and standard medical care.
- Studies have shown that yoga can be helpful for low back pain in the short term and may also be helpful over longer periods of time.
- An evaluation of research on herbal products for low back pain found preliminary evidence that devil's claw and white willow bark, taken orally (by mouth), may be helpful for back pain. Cayenne, comfrey, Brazilian arnica, and lavender essential oil may be helpful when used topically (applied to the skin).
- Studies of prolotherapy (a treatment involving repeated injections of irritant solutions) for low-back pain have had inconsistent results.

Osteoarthritis

- A combined analysis of data from several studies indicated that acupuncture can be helpful and a reasonable option to consider for osteoarthritis pain. After that analysis was completed, a Australian study showed that both needle and laser acupuncture were modestly better than no treatment at relieving knee pain from osteoarthritis but not better than simulated (sham) laser acupuncture. These results generally agree with previous studies, which showed that acupuncture is consistently better than no treatment but not necessarily better than simulated acupuncture at relieving osteoarthritis pain.
- A small amount of research suggests that massage may help reduce osteoarthritis symptoms.
- Tai chi may improve pain in people with knee osteoarthritis. Qi gong may have similar benefits, but little research has been done on it.
- It's uncertain whether yoga is helpful for osteoarthritis.
- Studies of glucosamine, chondroitin, and S-adenosyl-L-methionine (SAMe) for knee osteoarthritis pain have had conflicting results.
- There isn't enough research on dimethyl sulfoxide (DMSO) or methylsulfonylmethane (MSM) for osteoarthritis pain to allow conclusions to be reached.

Rheumatoid Arthritis

- The amount of research on mind and body practices for rheumatoid arthritis pain is too small for conclusions to be reached about their effectiveness.
- Dietary supplements containing omega-3 fatty acids, gamma-linolenic acid (GLA), or the herb thunder god vine may help relieve rheumatoid arthritis symptoms.

> Thunder god vine is a perennial grown in China and Taiwan. It has been used for hundreds of years in traditional Chinese medicine to treat swelling caused by inflammation. Currently, thunder god vine is used orally (by mouth) as a dietary supplement for autoimmune diseases, such as rheumatoid arthritis (RA), multiple sclerosis (MS), and lupus. It is also used topically for rheumatoid arthritis. Extracts are prepared from the roots of thunder god vine.
>
> *(Source: "Thunder God Vine," National Center for Complementary and Integrative Health (NCCIH).)*

Headache

- A combined analysis of data from several studies indicates that acupuncture can be helpful and a reasonable option to consider for headache pain. How acupuncture works to relieve pain is unclear. Current evidence suggests that many factors—like expectation and belief—that are unrelated to acupuncture needling may play important roles in the beneficial effects of acupuncture on pain.
- Because the evidence is limited or inconsistent, it's uncertain whether biofeedback, massage, relaxation techniques, spinal manipulation, and tai chi are helpful for headaches.
- *Guidelines* from the American Academy of Neurology (AAN) and the American Headache Society (AHS) classify butterbur as effective; feverfew, magnesium, and riboflavin as probably effective; and coenzyme Q10 as possibly effective for preventing migraines.

Neck Pain

- Acupuncture hasn't been studied as extensively for neck pain as for some other conditions. A large study in Germany found that people who received acupuncture for neck pain had better pain relief than those who didn't receive acupuncture. Several studies have compared actual acupuncture with simulated acupuncture, but the amount of research is limited. No current guidelines recommend acupuncture for neck pain.

- A review of studies performed in the United States found that massage therapy may provide short-term relief from neck pain, especially if massage sessions are relatively lengthy and frequent.
- Spinal manipulation may be helpful for neck pain.

Fibromyalgia

- It's uncertain whether acupuncture is helpful for fibromyalgia pain.
- Although some studies of tai chi, yoga, mindfulness, and biofeedback for fibromyalgia symptoms have had promising results, the evidence is too limited to allow definite conclusions to be reached about whether these approaches are helpful.
- There is insufficient evidence that any natural products can relieve fibromyalgia pain, with the possible exception of vitamin D supplements, which may reduce pain in people with fibromyalgia who have low vitamin D levels.
- Studies of homeopathy have not demonstrated that it is beneficial for fibromyalgia.

Irritable Bowel Syndrome (IBS)

- Although no complementary health approach has definitively been shown to be helpful for IBS, some research results for hypnotherapy and probiotics have been promising.
- There's only weak evidence supporting the idea that peppermint oil might be helpful for irritable bowel symptoms.
- Studies of acupuncture for IBS have not found actual acupuncture to be more helpful than simulated acupuncture.

Other Types Of Pain

- Various complementary approaches have been studied for other types of chronic pain, such as facial pain, nerve pain, chronic pelvic pain, elbow pain, pain associated with endometriosis, carpal tunnel syndrome, pain associated with gout, and cancer pain. There's promising evidence that some complementary approaches may be helpful for some of these types of pain, but the evidence is insufficient to clearly establish their effectiveness.

Other Complementary Approaches

- There is a lack of high-quality research to definitively evaluate whether Reiki is of value for pain relief.
- Although static magnets are widely marketed for pain control, the evidence does not support their use.

What The Science Says About Safety And Side Effects

As with any treatment, it's important to consider safety before using complementary health approaches. Safety depends on the specific approach and on the health of the person using it. If you're considering or using a complementary approach for pain, check with your healthcare providers to make sure it's safe for you.

Safety Of Mind And Body Approaches

- Mind and body approaches, such as acupuncture, hypnosis, massage therapy, mindfulness/meditation, relaxation techniques, spinal manipulation, tai chi/qi gong, and yoga, are generally safe for healthy people if they're performed appropriately.
  - People with medical conditions and pregnant women may need to modify or avoid some mind and body practices.
  - Like other forms of exercise, mind and body practices that involve movement, such as tai chi and yoga, can cause sore muscles and may involve some risk of injury.
  - It's important for practitioners and teachers of mind and body practices to be properly qualified and to follow appropriate safety precautions.

Safety Of Natural Products

- "Natural" doesn't always mean "safe." Some natural products (dietary supplements) may have side effects and may interact with medications.
- The U.S. Food and Drug Administration (FDA) has warned the public about several dietary supplements promoted for arthritis or pain that were tainted with prescription drugs.

Chapter 57

Asthma And Complementary Health Practices

Asthma is a chronic disease that affects your airways. Your airways are tubes that carry air in and out of your lungs. If you have asthma, the inside walls of your airways become sore and swollen. That makes them very sensitive, and they may react strongly to things that you are allergic to or find irritating. When your airways react, they get narrower and your lungs get less air.

Symptoms of asthma include:

- Wheezing
- Coughing, especially early in the morning or at night
- Chest tightness
- Shortness of breath

Not all people who have asthma have these symptoms. Having these symptoms doesn't always mean that you have asthma. Your doctor will diagnose asthma based on lung function tests, your medical history, and a physical exam. You may also have allergy tests.

When your asthma symptoms become worse than usual, it's called an asthma attack. Severe asthma attacks may require emergency care, and they can be fatal.

About This Chapter: Text in this chapter begins with excerpts from "Asthma," MedlinePlus, National Institutes of Health (NIH), January 2, 2017; Text under the heading "Treatment For Asthma" is excerpted from "Asthma: In Depth," National Center for Complementary and Integrative Health (NCCIH), April 2013. Reviewed January 2018; Text under the heading "Asthma And Complementary Health Practices" is excerpted from "4 Tips: Asthma And Complementary Health Practices," National Center for Complementary and Integrative Health (NCCIH), September 24, 2017.

Asthma is treated with two kinds of medicines:

1. Quick-relief medicines to stop asthma symptoms, and
2. Long-term control medicines to prevent symptoms.

Treatment For Asthma

More than 24 million people in the United States have been diagnosed with asthma, including approximately 7 million children. It is not known why some people develop asthma, but the tendency runs in families and the chance of having the disease appears to be increasing, especially among children.

Conventional treatment for asthma focuses on preventing attacks and relieving symptoms once an attack is underway. Prevention may include avoiding "asthma triggers" (the things that can set off or worsen symptoms) or taking medicine every day to prevent symptoms.

Once an asthma attack is underway, quick-relief medications may be used to relax muscles around the airways and open up airways so air can flow through them. Prevention techniques are generally preferred over quick-relief medications.

Asthma And Complementary Health Practices

Asthma is a chronic lung disease that affects people of all ages. It causes episodes of wheezing, coughing, shortness of breath, and chest tightness. Although there is no cure, most people are able to control their asthma with conventional therapies and by avoiding the substances that can set off asthma attacks. Even so, some people turn to complementary health practices such as acupuncture, breathing exercises, and herbal supplements in their efforts to relieve symptoms.

If you're thinking about complementary health practices for asthma, here's what you need to know: There is not enough evidence to support the use of any complementary health practices for the relief of asthma symptoms.

1. At this point, there is little evidence that acupuncture is an effective treatment for asthma. Although a few studies showed some reduction in medication use and improvements in symptoms and quality of life, most of the research showed no difference between real acupuncture and sham (fake) acupuncture on asthma symptoms.
2. A review of research on specific breathing techniques—the Papworth Method and Buteyko Breathing Technique—found a trend toward improvement in asthma

symptoms but not enough evidence to draw reliable conclusions. In spite of increasing patient interest in certain breathing exercises to help with symptoms like hyperventilation and to regulate breathing, there isn't solid evidence to support its use.

3. There is little or no evidence to support the use of herbs or dietary supplements for asthma. Some conventional treatments for asthma have their roots in herbal preparations: for example, the bronchodilator theophylline is found in tea leaves, and ephedrine (also a bronchodilator) is a compound in the traditional Chinese herb ma huang (ephedra*).
4. Researchers have found little or no evidence of benefit for the relief of asthma symptoms when they studied other herbs and dietary supplements such as boswellia, tylophora indica, magnesium supplements, omega-3 fatty acids, Radix glycyrrhizae, vitamin C, and butterbur.

Magnesium Supplements May Benefit People With Asthma

Research supported by National Center for Complementary and Integrative Health (NCCIH) and published in the *Journal of Asthma* provides additional evidence that adults with mild-to-moderate asthma may benefit from taking magnesium supplements. The researchers found that those who took magnesium experienced significant improvement in lung activity and the ability to move air in and out of their lungs. Those taking magnesium also reported other improvements in asthma control and quality of life compared with people who received placebo.

(Source: "Magnesium Supplements May Benefit People With Asthma," National Center for Complementary and Integrative Health (NCCIH).)

**In 2004, the U.S. Food and Drug Administration (FDA) banned the U.S. sale of dietary supplements containing ephedra. The FDA found that these supplements had an unreasonable risk of injury or illness—particularly cardiovascular complications—and a risk of death.*

Chapter 58

CAM Therapies For Cold And Flu

Flu And Cold

Each year, Americans get more than 1 billion colds, and between 5 and 20 percent of Americans get the flu. The two diseases have some symptoms in common, and both are caused by viruses. However, they are different conditions, and the flu is more severe. Unlike the flu, colds generally don't cause serious complications, such as pneumonia, or lead to hospitalization.

No vaccine can protect you against the common cold, but vaccines can protect you against the flu. Everyone over the age of 6 months should be vaccinated against the flu each year. Vaccination is the best protection against getting the flu. Prescription antiviral drugs may be used to treat the flu in people who are very ill or who are at high risk of flu complications. They're not a substitute for getting vaccinated. Vaccination is the first line of defense against the flu; antivirals are the second. If you think you've caught the flu, you may want to check with your healthcare provider to see whether antiviral medicine is appropriate for you. Call promptly. The drugs work best if they're used early in the illness.

What The Science Says About Complementary Health Approaches For The Flu

No complementary approach has been shown to prevent the flu or relieve flu symptoms.

Complementary approaches that have been studied for the flu include the following. In all instances, there's not enough evidence to show whether the approach is helpful.

About This Chapter: This chapter includes text excerpted from "Flu And Colds: In Depth," National Center for Complementary and Integrative Health (NCCIH), November 2016.

- American ginseng
- Chinese herbal medicines
- Echinacea
- Elderberry
- Green tea
- Oscillococcinum
- Vitamin C
- Vitamin D

What The Science Says About Complementary Health Approaches For Colds

The following complementary health approaches have been studied for colds:

American Ginseng

- Several studies have evaluated the use of American ginseng *(Panax quinquefolius)* to prevent colds. An evaluation of these studies concluded that the herb has not been shown to reduce the number of colds that people catch, although it may shorten the length of colds. The researchers who conducted the evaluation concluded that there was insufficient evidence to support the use of American ginseng for preventing colds.
- Taking American ginseng in an effort to prevent colds means taking it for prolonged periods of time. However, little is known about the herb's long-term safety. American ginseng may interact with the anticoagulant (blood thinning) drug warfarin.

Echinacea

- At least 24 studies have tested echinacea to see whether it can prevent colds or relieve cold symptoms. A comprehensive assessment of this research concluded that echinacea hasn't been convincingly shown to be beneficial. However, at least some echinacea products might have a weak effect.
- One reason why it's hard to reach definite conclusions about this herb is that echinacea products vary greatly. They may contain different species (types) of the plant and be made from different plant parts (the above-ground parts, the root, or both). They also

may be manufactured in different ways, and some products contain other ingredients in addition to echinacea. Research findings on one echinacea product may not apply to other products.

- Few side effects have been reported in studies of echinacea. However, some people are allergic to this herb, and in one study in children, taking echinacea was linked to an increase in rashes.

> There are nine known species of echinacea, all of which are native to North America. They were used by Native Americans of the Great Plains region as traditional medicines.
>
> Echinacea is used as a dietary supplement for the common cold and other infections, based on the idea that it might stimulate the immune system to more effectively fight infection. Echinacea preparations have been used topically (applied to the skin) for wounds and skin problems.
>
> The roots and above-ground parts of the echinacea plant are used fresh or dried to make teas, squeezed (expressed) juice, extracts, capsules and tablets, and preparations for external use. Several species of echinacea, most commonly *Echinacea purpurea* or *Echinacea angustifolia*, may be included in dietary supplements.
>
> *(Source: "Echinacea," National Center for Complementary and Integrative Health (NCCIH).)*

Garlic

- An evaluation of the research on garlic concluded that there isn't enough evidence to show whether this herb can help prevent colds or relieve their symptoms.
- Garlic can cause bad breath, body odor, and other side effects. Because garlic may interact with anticoagulant drugs (blood thinners), people who take these drugs should consult their healthcare providers before taking garlic.

Honey

- Honey's traditional reputation as a cough remedy has some science to back it up. A small amount of research suggests that honey may help to decrease nighttime coughing in children.
- Honey should never be given to infants under the age of 1 year because it may contain spores of the bacterium that causes infant botulism. Honey is considered safe for older children.

Meditation

- Meditation is generally considered to be safe for healthy people. However, there have been reports that it might worsen symptoms in people with certain chronic physical or mental health problems. If you have an ongoing health issue, talk with your healthcare provider before starting meditation.

Probiotics

- An evaluation of 13 studies found some evidence suggesting that probiotics might reduce the number of colds or other upper respiratory tract infections that people catch and the length of the illnesses, but the quality of the evidence was low or very low.
- In people who are generally healthy, probiotics have a good safety record. Side effects, if they occur at all, usually consist only of mild digestive symptoms such as gas. However, information on the long-term safety of probiotics is limited, and safety may differ from one type of probiotic to another. Probiotics have been linked to severe side effects, such as dangerous infections, in people with serious underlying medical problems.

Saline Nasal Irrigation

- Saline nasal irrigation means rinsing your nose and sinuses with salt water. People may do this with a neti pot (a device that comes from the Ayurvedic tradition) or with other devices, such as bottles, sprays, pumps, or nebulizers. Saline nasal irrigation may be used for sinus congestion, allergies, or colds.
- There's limited evidence that saline nasal irrigation can help relieve cold symptoms. Studies of this technique have been too small to allow researchers to reach definite conclusions.
- Saline nasal irrigation used to be considered safe, with only minor side effects such as nasal discomfort or irritation. However, a severe disease caused by an amoeba (a type of microorganism) was linked to nasal irrigation with tap water. The U.S. Food and Drug Administration (FDA) has warned that tap water that is not filtered, treated, or processed in specific ways is not safe for use in nasal rinsing devices and has explained how to use and clean these devices safely.

Vitamin C

- An evaluation of the large amount of research done on vitamin C and colds (29 studies involving more than 11,000 people) concluded that taking vitamin C doesn't prevent colds in the general population and shortens colds only slightly. Taking vitamin C only after you start to feel cold symptoms doesn't affect the length or severity of the cold.

- Unlike the situation in the general population, vitamin C does seem to reduce the number of colds in people exposed to short periods of extreme physical stress (such as marathon runners and skiers). In studies of these groups, taking vitamin C cut the number of colds in half.
- Taking too much vitamin C can cause diarrhea, nausea, and stomach cramps. People with the iron storage disease hemochromatosis should avoid high doses of vitamin C. People who are being treated for cancer or taking cholesterol-lowering medications should talk with their healthcare providers before taking vitamin C supplements.

Zinc

- Zinc has been used for colds in forms that are taken orally (by mouth), such as lozenges, tablets, or syrup, or used intranasally (in the nose), such as swabs or gels.
- **Oral Zinc**
    - An evaluation of 17 studies of various types of zinc lozenges, tablets, or syrup found that zinc can reduce the duration of colds.
    - Some participants in studies that tested zinc for cold reported that the zinc caused a bad taste or nausea.
    - Long-term use of high doses of zinc can cause low copper levels, reduced immunity, and low levels of high-density lipoproteins (HDL) cholesterol (the "good" cholesterol). Zinc may interact with drugs, including antibiotics and penicillamine (a drug used to treat rheumatoid arthritis).
- **Intranasal Zinc**
    - The use of zinc products inside the nose, such as gels or swabs, may cause loss of the sense of smell, which may be long-lasting or permanent. In 2009, the FDA warned consumers to stop using several intranasal zinc products marketed as cold remedies because of this risk.
    - Prior to the warnings about effects on the sense of smell, a few studies of intranasal zinc had suggested a possible benefit against cold symptoms. However, the risk of a serious and lasting side effect outweighs any possible benefit in the treatment of a minor illness.

Other Complementary Approaches

In addition to the complementary approaches described above, several other approaches have been studied for colds. In all instances, there is insufficient evidence to show whether these approaches help to prevent colds or relieve cold symptoms.

- Andrographis (*Andrographis paniculata*)
- Chinese herbal medicines
- Green tea
- Guided imagery
- Hydrotherapy
- Vitamin D
- Vitamin E

Chapter 59

Diabetes And CAM

About Diabetes

- Diabetes is a disease that occurs when your blood glucose, also called blood sugar, is too high. It can lead to serious health problems if it's not managed well.
- Taking insulin or other diabetes medicine is often key to treating diabetes, along with making healthy food choices and being physically active.
- Your healthcare providers can show you how to control your diabetes and track your success.
- There are three types of diabetes—type 1, type 2, and gestational. All three involve problems with how your body responds to the hormone insulin. Food supplies your body with glucose, a sugar and the main fuel for our bodies. To use glucose, your body needs insulin. If you have type 1 diabetes your body is producing little or no insulin. If you have type 2 your body makes insulin but doesn't respond to it normally. Gestational diabetes affects only pregnant women. It usually goes away after birth, but it increases the mother's risk of developing diabetes later in life.
- About 95 percent of people diagnosed with diabetes have type 2. People with type 1, which is usually diagnosed in childhood or early adulthood, must take insulin to survive.

Kidney disease has been linked to using some dietary supplements. This is of particular concern for people with diabetes, since diabetes is the leading cause of kidney failure in the

About This Chapter: This chapter includes text excerpted from "Diabetes And Dietary Supplements: In Depth," National Center for Complementary and Integrative Health (NCCIH), July 24, 2017.

United States. If you have or are at risk for kidney disease, a healthcare provider should closely monitor your use of supplements.

What The Science Says About The Effectiveness And Safety Of Dietary Supplements For Diabetes

Alpha-Lipoic Acid

Alpha-lipoic acid is an antioxidant (a substance that may protect against cell damage) being studied for its effect on complications of diabetes, including macular edema, an eye condition that causes blurred vision; unhealthy cholesterol levels; and poor insulin sensitivity. Two studies of about 570 patients didn't find that the supplement helped with conditions related to diabetes.

Safety

High doses of alpha-lipoic acid supplements can cause stomach problems.

Chromium

Found in many foods, chromium is an essential trace mineral. If you have too little chromium in your diet, your body can't use glucose efficiently.

- Studies have found few or no benefits of chromium supplements for controlling diabetes or reducing the risk of developing it. Taking chromium supplements, along with conventional care, improved blood sugar control in people with diabetes (primarily type 2) who had poor blood sugar control, a review concluded; however, the improvement was very small. The review included 25 studies with about 1,600 participants.

Safety

Chromium supplements may cause stomach pain and bloating, and there have been a few reports of kidney damage, muscular problems, and skin reactions following large doses. The effects of taking chromium long term haven't been well investigated.

Herbal Supplements

Researchers don't have reliable evidence that any herbal supplements can help to control diabetes or its complications.

- There are no clear benefits of cinnamon for people with diabetes.

- Other herbal supplements studied for diabetes include bitter melon, Chinese herbal medicines, fenugreek, ginseng, milk thistle, selenium, and sweet potato. Studies haven't proven that any of these are effective, and some may have side effects.

Safety

Researchers have little conclusive information on the safety of herbal supplements for people with diabetes.

- Cassia cinnamon, the most common type of cinnamon sold in the United States and Canada, contains varying amounts of a chemical called coumarin, which might cause or worsen liver disease. In most cases, cassia cinnamon doesn't have enough coumarin to make you sick. However, for some people, such as those with liver disease, taking a large amount of cassia cinnamon might worsen their condition.
- Using herbs such as St. John's wort, prickly pear cactus, aloe, or ginseng with conventional diabetes drugs can cause unwanted side effects.

Magnesium

Found in many foods, including in high amounts in bran cereal, certain seeds and nuts, and spinach, magnesium is essential to the body's ability to process glucose.

- Magnesium deficiency may increase the risk of developing diabetes. A number of studies have looked at whether taking magnesium supplements helps people who have diabetes or who are at risk of developing it. However, the studies are generally small and their results aren't conclusive.

Safety

Large doses of magnesium in supplements can cause diarrhea and abdominal cramping. Very large doses—more than 5,000 mg per day—can be deadly.

Omega-3s

- Taking omega-3 supplements, such as fish oil, hasn't been shown to help people who have diabetes control their blood sugar levels. Research on whether eating fish lowers your risk of getting diabetes is generally negative. However, the effect of eating fish may depend on what type of fish you eat, among other factors.
- Studies on the effects of eating fish have had conflicting results, two research reviews with hundreds of thousands of participants showed. Some research from the United

States and Europe found that people who ate more fish had a higher incidence of diabetes. Research from Asia and Australia found the opposite—eating more fish was associated with a lower risk of diabetes. There's no strong evidence explaining these differences.

- Taking omega-3 supplements doesn't help protect against heart disease in people who have or are at risk of having diabetes, an American Heart Association (AHA) science advisory, based on 5 studies with more than 10,000 participants, stated in 2017. However, it's unclear whether people who have both diabetes and a high risk of developing heart disease would benefit from taking omega-3 supplements.

Safety

Omega-3 supplements don't usually have side effects. When side effects do occur, they typically consist of minor symptoms, such as bad breath, indigestion, or diarrhea. It may interact with drugs that affect blood clotting.

Vitamins

- Studies generally show that taking vitamin C doesn't improve blood sugar control or other conditions in people with diabetes. However, a 2017 research review of 22 studies with 937 participants found weak evidence that vitamin C helped with blood sugar in people with type 2 diabetes when they took it for longer than 30 days.
- Having low levels of vitamin D is associated with an increased risk of developing a metabolic disorder, such as type 2 diabetes, metabolic syndrome, or insulin resistance, studies and research reviews from the past 5 years have found. But taking vitamin D doesn't appear to help prevent diabetes or improve blood sugar levels for people with normal levels, prediabetes, or type 2 diabetes, a 2014 research review of 35 studies with 43,407 participants showed.

Safety

Taking too much vitamin D is dangerous and can cause nausea, constipation, weakness, kidney damage, disorientation, and problems with your heart rhythm. You're unlikely to get too much vitamin D from food or the sun.

Other Supplements

- The evidence is still very preliminary on how supplements or foods rich in polyphenols—antioxidants found in tea, coffee, wine, fruits, grains, and vegetables—might affect diabetes.

Healthy Behaviors: Key To Managing Your Diabetes

Diet

Develop a meal plan with help from your healthcare providers.

Physical Activity

Different types and even small amounts of physical activity can help you control diabetes. Physical activity lowers blood sugar, blood pressure, improves blood flow, and more. Talk with your healthcare provider before you start a new physical activity program.

Stay Safe When Blood Glucose Is High

If you have type 1 diabetes, avoid vigorous physical activity when you have ketones in your blood or urine. Ketones are chemicals your body might make when your blood glucose level is too high, a condition called hyperglycemia, and your insulin level is too low. If you are physically active when you have ketones in your blood or urine, your blood glucose level may go even higher. Ask your healthcare team what level of ketones are dangerous for you and how to test for them. Ketones are uncommon in people with type 2 diabetes.

(Source: "Diabetes Overview—Diabetes Diet, Eating, And Physical Activity," National Institute of Diabetes and Digestive and Kidney Diseases (NIDDK).)

What Do We Know About The Safety Of Dietary Supplements For Diabetes?

- Some dietary supplements have side effects, including interacting with diabetes treatments or increasing the risk of kidney problems.
- The U.S. Food and Drug Administration (FDA) is warning consumers not to buy illegally marketed, potentially dangerous products claiming to prevent, treat, or cure diabetes.
- It's very important not to replace proven conventional medical treatment for diabetes with an unproven health product or practice.

Chapter 60

Irritable Bowel Syndrome And Complementary Health Practices

What Is Irritable Bowel Syndrome (IBS)?

IBS is a chronic disorder that affects the large intestine and causes symptoms such as abdominal pain, cramping, constipation, and diarrhea. As many as one in five Americans have symptoms of IBS. The cause of IBS isn't well understood but stress, large meals, certain foods, and alcohol may trigger symptoms in people with this disorder.

What The Science Says About The Effectiveness Of Complementary Health Approaches For IBS

Some evidence is emerging that a few complementary health approaches may be helpful for IBS. However, the research is limited so researchers don't know for sure.

Mind And Body Practices For IBS

- **Acupuncture**
  - For easing the severity of IBS, actual acupuncture wasn't better than simulated acupuncture, a systematic review reported.
  - A clinical trial included in the review found that of the 230 participants with IBS, those who received either actual or simulated acupuncture did better than those who received no acupuncture.

About This Chapter: This chapter includes text excerpted from "Irritable Bowel Syndrome: In Depth," National Center for Complementary and Integrative Health (NCCIH), March 2015.

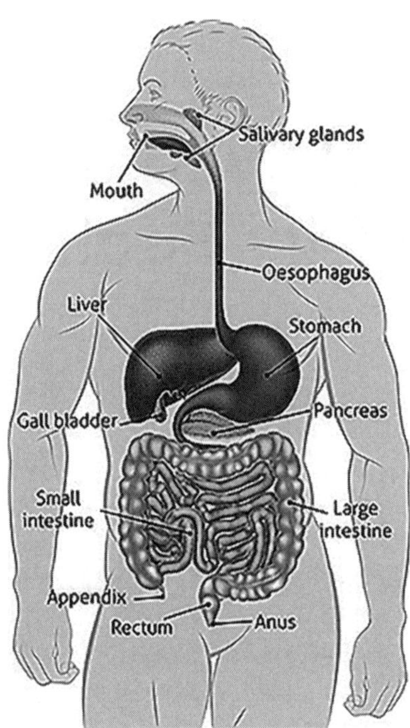

Figure 60.1. Inflammatory Bowel Disease (IBD)

IBD is a collection of inflammatory conditions of colon and small intestine.

(Source: "Inflammatory Bowel Disease (IBD): What Is It?" Centers for Disease Control and Prevention (CDC).)

- **Hypnotherapy (Hypnosis)**

  Researchers are studying gut-directed hypnotherapy (GDH), which focuses on improving bowel symptoms. Several IBS studies have found an association between hypnotherapy and long-term improvement in gastrointestinal symptoms, anxiety, depression, disability, and quality of life. The American College of Gastroenterology (ACG) stated in a paper that there is some evidence that hypnosis helps with IBS symptoms, but the research is very uncertain.

  - Just more than half of study participants who had 10 GDH sessions over 12 weeks felt better, compared with 25 percent of participants not assigned to undergo GDH, a 2013 study of 90 patients with IBS showed. The benefits lasted for at least 15 months. The non-GDH group had the same number of sessions of supportive talks with a physician who was trained in diseases related to stress and other factors.

- A research review suggested that children with IBS who underwent GDH had greater reductions in abdominal pain than children who received standard treatment. This was true whether the children underwent GDH with a therapist or listened to an audio recording. However, the result may not be reliable, as the researchers found only three small studies that met their standards.
- Many children and adolescents with mild IBS symptoms who get only reassurance from their healthcare provider improve over time.

- **Mindfulness Meditation Training**

  Some studies suggest that mindfulness training helps people with IBS, but there's not enough evidence to draw firm conclusions.

  - The ACG stated in a paper that the few studies that have looked at mindfulness meditation training for IBS found no significant effects. But the researchers noted that given the limited number of studies, they can't be sure it doesn't help. A review that included these and other studies concluded that mindfulness training improved IBS-associated pain and quality of life but not depression or anxiety. The amount of improvement was small.
  - A National Center for Complementary and Integrative Health (NCCIH)-supported clinical trial of 75 women with IBS showed that mindfulness training may decrease the severity of IBS symptoms, including psychological distress, compared to attending a support group. The benefits lasted for at least 3 months after the training ended.
  - Yoga. In a small NCCIH-supported study, young adults (18–26 years old) reported generally feeling better and having less pain, constipation, and nausea after completing a series of yoga classes, compared with a waitlist control group. They were still feeling better at the study's 2-month follow-up. There's too little evidence to draw conclusions about the effectiveness of meditation, relaxation training, and reflexology for IBS.

About Dietary Supplements For IBS

A variety of dietary supplements, many of which are Chinese herbs and herb combinations, have been investigated for IBS, but we can't draw any conclusions about them because of the poor quality of many of the studies.

- **Chinese herbs.** In a systematic review, a combination of Chinese herbs was associated with improved IBS symptoms, but extracts of three single herbs had no beneficial effects.

- **Peppermint oil.** Peppermint oil capsules may be modestly helpful in reducing several common symptoms of IBS, including abdominal pain and bloating. It's superior to placebo in improving IBS symptoms.
- **Probiotics.** Generally, probiotics improve IBS symptoms, bloating, and flatulence, the ACG stated in a 2014 paper. However, it noted that the quality of existing studies is limited. It's not possible to draw firm conclusions about specific probiotics for IBS in part because studies have used different species, strains, preparations, and doses.

Probiotics are live microorganisms, most often bacteria, that are similar to microorganisms you normally have in your digestive tract.

(Source: "Irritable Bowel Syndrome (IBS)," National Institute of Diabetes and Digestive and Kidney Diseases (NIDDK).)

Things To Consider

- Unproven products or practices should not be used to replace conventional treatments for IBS or as a reason to postpone seeing a healthcare provider about IBS symptoms or any other health problem.
- If you're considering a practitioner-provided complementary practice such as hypnotherapy or acupuncture, ask a trusted source (such as the healthcare provider who treats your IBS or a nearby hospital) to recommend a practitioner. Find out about the training and experience of any practitioner you're considering.
- Keep in mind that dietary supplements may interact with medications or other supplements and may contain ingredients not listed on the label. Your healthcare provider can advise you. If you're pregnant or nursing a child, or if you're considering giving a child a dietary supplement, it's especially important to consult your (or your child's) healthcare provider.
- Tell all of your healthcare providers about any complementary health approaches you use. Give them a full picture of what you do to manage your health. This will help ensure coordinated and safe care.

Chapter 61

Alternative, Complementary, And Traditional Medicine For HIV

Many people use complementary (sometimes known as alternative) health treatments to go along with the medical care they get from their doctor.

These therapies are called "complementary" therapies because usually they are used alongside the more standard medical care you receive (such as your doctor visits and the anti-HIV drugs you might be taking).

They are sometimes called "alternative" because they don't fit into the more mainstream, Western ways of looking at medicine and healthcare. These therapies may not fit in with what you usually think of as "healthcare."

Some common complementary therapies include:

- Physical (body) therapies, such as yoga, massage, and acupuncture
- Relaxation techniques, such as meditation and visualization
- Herbal medicine (from plants)

With most complementary therapies, your health is looked at from a holistic (or "whole picture") point of view. Think of your body as working as one big system. From a holistic viewpoint, everything you do—from what you eat to what you drink to how stressed you are—affects your health and well-being.

About This Chapter: This chapter includes text excerpted from "Alternative (Complementary) Therapies For HIV/AIDS," U.S. Department of Veterans Affairs (VA), August 9, 2016.

Do Alternative Therapies Work?

Healthy people use these kinds of therapies to try to make their immune systems stronger and to make themselves feel better in general. People who have diseases or illnesses, such as human immunodeficiency virus (HIV), use these therapies for the same reasons. They also can use these therapies to help deal with symptoms of the disease or side effects from the medicines that treat the disease.

Many people report positive results from using complementary therapies. In most cases, however, there is not enough research to tell if these treatments really help people with HIV.

If You Want To Try Complementary Treatments To Help You Cope With HIV/AIDS, Please Remember These Things:

- Always talk to your healthcare provider before you start any kind of treatment, even if you think it is safe.
- Just because something is "natural" (an herb, for example) doesn't mean that it is safe to take. Sometimes these products can interact with your HIV medicines or cause side effects on their own. St. John's wort, for example, decreases levels of some HIV medications in your blood.
- The federal government does not require that herbal remedies and dietary supplements be tested in the same way that standard medicines are tested before they are sold. Many of the treatments out there have not been studied as much as the HIV drugs you are taking. It is always a risk to take something or try something that hasn't been fully studied or researched.
- Be careful of treatments that claim to be "miracle cures"—ones that claim to cure human immunodeficiency virus (HIV)/acquired immune deficiency syndrome (AIDS). There are people out there who may try to trick you into buying an expensive product that doesn't work. Always do your research and ask your doctor for help.
- Complementary therapies are not substitutes for the treatment and drugs you receive from your doctor. Never stop taking your anti-HIV drugs just because you've started another therapy.
- The federal government is funding studies of how well some alternative therapies work to treat disease, so keep your eyes open for news about these studies.

Here you can read about some of the more common complementary therapies that people with HIV use. Sometimes these are used alone, but often they are used in combination with one another. For example, some people combine yoga with meditation.

Physical (Body) Therapies

Physical, or body, therapies include such activities as yoga, massage, and aromatherapy. These types of therapies focus on using a person's body and senses to promote healing and well-being. Here you can learn about examples of these types of therapies.

Yoga

Yoga is a set of exercises that people use to improve their fitness, reduce stress, and increase flexibility.

Yoga can involve breathing exercises, certain stretches and poses, and meditation.

Many people, including people with HIV, use yoga to reduce stress and to become more relaxed and calm. Some people think that yoga helps make them healthier in general, because it can make a person's body stronger.

If you would like to try yoga, talk to your healthcare provider. There are many different types of yoga and various classes you can take. You can also try out yoga by following a program on videotape.

Before you begin any kind of exercise program, always talk with your doctor.

Massage

Many people believe that massage therapy is an excellent way to deal with the stress and side effects that go along with having an illness, including HIV.

During massage therapy, a trained therapist moves and rubs your body tissues (such as your muscles). There are many kinds of massage therapy.

You can try massage therapy for reducing muscle and back pain, headaches, and soreness. Massages also can improve your blood flow (your circulation) and reduce tension. Some people think that massages might even make your immune system stronger.

If you are interested in learning more about massage, you should ask your doctor to recommend a trained therapist. Your doctor may have a list of trained massage therapists, so if you want to learn more about massage, ask.

Acupuncture

Acupuncture is part of a whole healing system known as traditional Chinese medicine. During acupuncture treatment, tiny needles (about as wide as a hair) are inserted into certain areas of a person's body. Most people say that they don't feel any pain at all from the needles.

Many people with HIV use acupuncture. Some people think that acupuncture can help treat symptoms of HIV and side effects from the medicine, like fatigue and stomach aches.

Some people say that acupuncture can be used to help with neuropathy (body pain caused by nerve damage from HIV or the medicines used to treat HIV).

Others report that acupuncture gives them more energy.

If you are interested in trying it out, ask your doctor to recommend an expert. At the end of this guide are links to websites where you can read more about the history of acupuncture and how it works.

Aromatherapy

Aromatherapy is based on the idea that certain smells can change the way you feel. The smells used in aromatherapy come from plant oils, and they can be inhaled (breathed in) or used in baths or massages.

People use aromatherapy to help them deal with stress or to help with fatigue. For example, some people report that lavender oil calms them down and helps them sleep better.

You can also ask friends or family if they've tried aromatherapy or know someone who has. At the end of this guide are links to websites where you can learn more about aromatherapy.

Please remember! The oils used in aromatherapy can be very strong and even harmful. Always talk with an expert before buying and using these oils yourself.

Relaxation Techniques

Relaxation therapies, such as meditation and visualization, focus on how a person's mind and imagination can promote overall health and well-being. In this section, you can read about some examples of how you can use relaxation therapies to reduce stress and relax.

Meditation

Meditation is a certain way of concentrating that allows your mind and body to become very relaxed. Meditation helps people to focus and be quiet.

There are many different forms of meditation. Most involve deep breathing and paying attention to your body and mind.

Sometimes people sit still and close their eyes to meditate. Meditation also can be casual. For instance, you can meditate when you are taking a walk or watching a sunrise.

People with HIV can use meditation to relax. It can help them deal with the stress that comes with any illness. Meditation can help you to calm down and focus if you are feeling overwhelmed.

If you are interested in learning more about meditation, you should ask your healthcare provider for more information. There may be meditation classes you can take. At the end of this guide are links to websites where you can learn more.

Visualization

Visualization is another method people use to feel more relaxed and less anxious. People who use visualization imagine that they are in a safe, relaxing place (such as the beach). Most of us use visualization without realizing it—for example, when researchers daydream or remember a fun, happy time in our lives.

Focusing on a safe, comfortable place can help you to feel less stress, and sometimes it can lessen the pain or side effects from HIV or the medicines you are taking.

You can ask your doctor where you can learn more about visualization. There are classes you can take, and there are self-help tapes that you can listen to that lead you through the process.

Herbal Medicine

Herbal medicines are substances that come from plants, and they work like standard medicine. They can be taken from all parts of a plant, including the roots, leaves, berries, and flowers.

People with HIV sometimes take these medicines to help deal with side effects from anti-HIV medicines or with symptoms from the illness.

An important note about St. John's wort: St. John's wort has become a popular herbal medicine for treating depression. It interacts with the liver and can change how some drugs work in your body, including some anti-HIV drugs (for example, protease inhibitors and Non-nucleoside reverse-transcriptase inhibitors (NNRTIs)). If you are taking antiviral drugs for your HIV, you should NOT take St. John's wort. Be sure you tell you doctor if you are using St. John's wort. You should also not take St. John's wort if you are taking other antidepressants.

- It is important to remember to always use herbs carefully. Learn the proper dosage and use. Don't take too much of anything.
- Always ask your doctor before taking anything new. Just because something is "natural" or "nondrug" doesn't mean that it is safe.
- Finally, learn about the possible side effects of an herbal therapy. Remember: Some herbs can interfere with your HIV medications.

Chapter 62

CAM For Hepatitis C

Hepatitis C is a liver disease caused by a virus. It's usually chronic (long-lasting), but most people don't have any symptoms until the virus causes liver damage, which can take 10 or more years to happen. Without medical treatment, chronic hepatitis C can eventually cause liver cancer or liver failure. Conventional medical treatments are available for chronic hepatitis C. Some people with hepatitis C also try complementary health approaches, especially dietary supplements.

Use Of Herbal Supplements And Other Complementary Approaches For Hepatitis C

Several herbal supplements have been studied for hepatitis C, and substantial numbers of people with hepatitis C have tried herbal supplements. For example, a survey of 1,145 participants in the HALT-C (Hepatitis C Antiviral Long-Term Treatment Against Cirrhosis) trial, a study supported by the National Institutes of Health (NIH), found that 23 percent of the participants were using herbal products. Although participants reported using many different herbal products, silymarin (milk thistle) was by far the most common.

What The Science Says

No dietary supplement has been shown to be effective for hepatitis C. This chapter summarizes what's known about the safety and effectiveness of milk thistle and some of the other dietary supplements studied for hepatitis C.

About This Chapter: This chapter includes text excerpted from "Hepatitis C: A Focus On Dietary Supplements," National Center for Complementary and Integrative Health (NCCIH), November 2014. Reviewed January 2018.

- **Milk thistle** (scientific name Silybum marianum) is a plant from the aster family. Silymarin is an active component of milk thistle believed to be responsible for the herb's health-related properties. Milk thistle has been used in Europe for treating liver disease and jaundice since the 16th century. In the United States, silymarin is the most popular dietary supplement taken by people with liver disease. However, two rigorously designed studies of silymarin in people with hepatitis C didn't show any benefit.
- A controlled clinical trial, co-funded by National Center for Complementary and Integrative Health (NCCIH) and National Institute of Diabetes and Digestive and Kidney Diseases (NIDDK), showed that two higher-than-usual doses of silymarin were no better than placebo in reducing the high blood levels of an enzyme that indicates liver damage. In the study, 154 people who hadn't responded to standard antiviral treatment for chronic hepatitis C were randomly assigned to receive 420 mg of silymarin, 700 mg of silymarin, or placebo three times per day for 24 weeks. At the end of the treatment period, blood levels of the enzyme were similar in all three groups.
- Results of the HALT-C study mentioned above suggested that silymarin use by hepatitis C patients was associated with fewer and milder symptoms of liver disease and somewhat better quality of life, but there was no change in virus activity or liver inflammation. The researchers emphasized that this was a retrospective study (one that examined the medical and lifestyle histories of the participants). Its finding of improved quality of life in patients taking silymarin wasn't confirmed in the more rigorous study described above.

Safety. Available evidence from clinical trials in people with liver disease suggests that milk thistle is generally well tolerated. Side effects can include a laxative effect, nausea, diarrhea, abdominal bloating and pain, and occasional allergic reactions. In NIH-funded studies of silymarin in people with hepatitis C, the frequency of side effects was similar in people taking silymarin and those taking placebos. However, these studies were not large enough to show with certainty that silymarin is safe for people with chronic hepatitis C.

Other supplements have been studied for hepatitis C, but overall, no benefits have been clearly demonstrated. These supplements include the following:

- **Probiotics** are live microorganisms that are intended to have a health benefit when consumed. Research hasn't produced any clear evidence that probiotics are helpful in people with hepatitis C. Most people can use probiotics without experiencing any side effects—or with only mild gastrointestinal (GI) side effects such as intestinal gas—but there have been some case reports of serious adverse effects in people with underlying serious health conditions.

- Preliminary studies, most of which were conducted outside the United States, have examined the use of **zinc** for hepatitis C. Zinc supplements might help to correct zinc deficiencies associated with hepatitis C or reduce some symptoms, but the evidence for these possible benefits is limited. Zinc is generally considered to be safe when used appropriately, but it can be toxic if taken in excessive amounts.
- A few preliminary studies have looked at the effects of combining supplements such as lactoferrin, S-adenosyl-L-methionine (SAMe), or zinc with conventional drug therapy for hepatitis C. The evidence isn't sufficient to draw clear conclusions about benefit or safety.
- Glycyrrhizin—a compound found in licorice root—has been tested in a few clinical trials in hepatitis C patients, but there's currently not enough evidence to determine if it's helpful. In large amounts, glycyrrhizin or licorice can be dangerous in people with a history of hypertension (high blood pressure), kidney failure, or cardiovascular diseases (CVD).
- Preliminary studies have examined the potential of the following products for treating chronic hepatitis C: TJ-108 (a mixture of herbs used in Japanese Kampo medicine), schisandra, oxymatrine (an extract from the sophora root), and thymus extract. The limited research on these products hasn't produced convincing evidence that they're helpful for hepatitis C.
- Colloidal silver has been suggested as a treatment for hepatitis C, but there's currently no research to support its use for this purpose. Colloidal silver is known to cause serious side effects, including a permanent bluish discoloration of the skin called argyria.

If You're Considering Taking A Dietary Supplement For Hepatitis C

- Do not use any complementary health approach to replace conventional treatments for hepatitis C or as a reason to postpone seeing your healthcare provider about any medical problem.
- Be aware that dietary supplements may have side effects or interact with conventional medical treatments.

If you are considering any dietary supplement for hepatitis C, here are some things you should know.

1. No dietary supplement has been shown to be effective for hepatitis C or its complications.
2. The results of research supported by the NIH have shown that silymarin, the active extract of milk thistle and the most popular complementary health product taken by people with liver disease, was no more effective than placebo in people with hepatitis C.
3. Research on other dietary supplements for hepatitis C, such as zinc, licorice root (or its extract glycyrrhizin), SAMe, and lactoferrin, is in its early stages, and no firm conclusions can be reached about the potential effectiveness of these supplements.
4. Colloidal silver is sometimes promoted for treating hepatitis C, but is not safe. Colloidal silver can cause irreversible side effects, including a permanent bluish discoloration of the skin.
5. Check with your healthcare provider before using any dietary supplement to make sure that it is safe for you and compatible with any medical treatment that you are receiving for hepatitis C or any other health problem.

(Source: "5 Things You Should Know About Dietary Supplements For Hepatitis C," National Center for Complementary and Integrative Health (NCCIH).)

Chapter 63

CAM Therapies In Behavioral Health

What Is The Appeal Of Complementary Health Approaches For Behavioral Health Treatment?

For a variety of reasons, complementary health approaches can be especially appealing to behavioral health clients. Individuals who have not been successful with a particular conventional treatment maybe curious about trying complementary therapies as adjuncts or treatment alternatives. Or, such individuals may hope that augmenting conventional treatment will enhance their recovery. Some clients may have a lifestyle preference for products and healing systems they perceive as natural, want to avoid medication side effects, or appreciate the hands-on care they receive from a complementary health practitioner. From the standpoint of the behavioral health treatment program, offering a complementary therapy that is culturally relevant or popular in the community may attract prospective clients to the program's conventional treatment offerings and support retention. Some practices, such as meditation or movement-based therapies, may help clients gain self-efficacy skills. Complementary practices offered to groups may also enhance clients' socialization skills and support systems.

About This Chapter: Text beginning with the heading "What Is The Appeal Of Complementary Health Approaches For Behavioral Health Treatment?" is excerpted from "Advisory," Substance Abuse and Mental Health Services Administration (SAMHSA), 2015; Text under the heading "What Can Complementary And Alternative Medicine (CAM) Do For Anxiety?" is excerpted from "Safe Use Of Complementary Health Products And Practices For Anxiety," MedlinePlus, National Institutes of Health (NIH), 2015.

How Effective Are Complementary Health Approaches?

Complementary health approaches have been insufficiently studied compared with conventional treatments. Many of the studies that have been conducted lack one or more features of the randomized controlled trial (RCT), which is the gold standard for evaluating biomedical or behavioral interventions. An RCT compares a treatment with a different treatment or with a placebo and randomly assigns subjects to experimental and control (comparison) groups. RCTs are often blinded (that is, the subjects or the scientists administering the experiment, or both, do not know which treatment each subject is receiving) and, ideally, include sample sizes large enough for study results to achieve statistical significance. A well-designed RCT seeks to account for all possible variables that may influence the study results

These features of the RCT can present challenges when assessing complementary practices. For example, some complementary practices involve multiple components (e.g., movement combined with meditation and deep breathing); teasing apart the effects of each component adds to the already considerable amount of time, funds, and labor required to conduct an RCT. Also, when studying interventions such as yoga or acupuncture, it is often not feasible to blind study participants and those administering the intervention. Yet another challenge is that complementary health practitioners typically customize the treatment to the individual. For purposes of an RCT, however, the intervention must be standardized, which can make a study's results less relevant to real-world application. The challenges of evaluating complementary health approaches through well-designed RCTs are prompting health researchers to explore alternative trial designs. Another challenge in evaluating the efficacy of complementary health approaches is the ongoing debate over the value of the placebo effect. Evidence on a variety of complementary practices indicates that positive effects that occur may be attributable not to the treatment itself, but rather to the interaction between the complementary health practitioner and the patient, the patient's beliefs and expectations about the treatment, and the setting and cultural context in which it is provided. Evidence that the placebo effect may play a potentially significant role in some complementary therapies has led some researchers to label complementary health approaches as "placebos." However, some researchers claim that the placebo effect is a powerful force that can be effectively harnessed through complementary health approaches to facilitate the body's ability to heal itself. The task of helping clients make informed, evidence-based decisions about complementary health approaches is complicated by—as just described—the lack of convincing data, questions about the most appropriate means of evaluating these practices, and the unresolved controversy over the role of placebo in treatment.

Presented below are summaries of the existing evidence on selected complementary health approaches for mental or substance use disorders, as provided by systematic reviews and meta-analyses.

Acupuncture

Acupuncture is a low-risk, low-cost therapy that, based on anecdotal evidence, can relieve physical withdrawal symptoms, help with relaxation, and suppress cravings for drugs and alcohol. A small percentage of substance abuse treatment programs—4.4 percent—offer acupuncture as an adjunct therapy. Some systematic reviews have focused specifically on acupuncture for treatment of disorders involving opioids, alcohol, and cocaine. These reviews did not find evidence of efficacy, and the authors have concluded that more research is needed. A 2009 review of clinical trials found some evidence for acupuncture's effectiveness with opioid withdrawal but not for treatment of other conditions such as alcohol withdrawal, nicotine relapse prevention, or cocaine dependence. A 2013 review of 48 RCTs testing acupuncture for use with patients who had alcohol, cocaine, nicotine, or opioid dependence concluded that nearly half of the clinical trials reviewed had at least one positive result (e.g., on craving), indicating that different types of acupuncture may have beneficial effects at different points in the withdrawal and recovery process. A substantial number of studies have been done on acupuncture as a treatment for mental disorders. A review published by the American Psychiatric Association's Task Force on Complementary and Alternative Medicine concluded that the data do not suggest that acupuncture is effective in treating major depressive disorder.

Mindfulness Meditation

An increasing amount of research has focused on mindfulness meditation, with 477 articles published in academic journals in 2012 alone. In a systematic review of 14 randomized and 10 nonrandomized controlled trials, the authors found evidence that mindfulness-based interventions can reduce consumption of substances of abuse when compared with various controls, and they found preliminary evidence that the interventions can reduce cravings.

Movement Therapies

For the treatment of mental or substance use disorders, exercise is theorized to provide social and psychological benefits by increasing socialization, improving emotional regulation, decreasing sensitivity to anxiety, and improving stress management. It is also postulated that because exercise triggers neurological effects similar to those produced by opioid drugs, exercise may serve as a substitute for substance use.

Exercise to promote physical, mental, emotional, or spiritual health is called movement therapy. Some studies have investigated movement therapies in relation to specific mental or substance use disorders. A 2013 meta-analysis of 37 RCTs found that exercise is moderately more effective than no therapy or a control intervention for reducing symptoms of depression. A 2011 meta-analysis of 10 RCTs found that yoga-based interventions have a statistically significant effect when used as an adjunct for treating severe mental illness, especially when current treatment modalities are inadequate or have adverse effects (e.g., weight gain, cardiovascular disease). A 2014 review of eight studies on yoga for treatment of addictions reported that seven of those studies showed positive effects; the article authors concluded that the results are "encouraging but inconclusive" because of methodological limitations.

Although evidence of exercise's effect on mental and substance use disorders is inconclusive, the benefits of routine physical exercise for overall health, wellness, and quality of life are well documented. At the least, exercise can be a helpful adjunct therapy to behavioral health treatment, and clients may benefit from participation in a movement-based complementary practice such as yoga, Pilates, or tai chi. A doctor's guidance on appropriate types of exercise or movement therapy is advised for clients who are pregnant, have a specific medical condition (e.g., multiple sclerosis, back injury, osteoporosis), or have not exercised in a long time.

Natural Products

Of the many dietary supplements marketed to consumers as having mental health benefits, two of the most popular are omega-3 supplements and SAMe (S-adenosyl-L-methionine). Some omega-3 fatty acids are essential nutrients obtained from food sources such as fatty fish and certain plants such as flax. SAMe is a chemical that is naturally found in almost all tissues in the body. Table 63.1 provides evidence of effectiveness and cautions for both of these products. Many herbal products are also marketed to consumers for treatment of mental disorders. Table 63.1 lists two examples, kava and St. John's wort. Among the many other botanicals marketed as treatments for mental health conditions are brook mint for anxiety or insomnia, chamomile for insomnia, lavender for anxiety or insomnia, linden for insomnia and nervous tension, passion flower for insomnia and anxiety, and valerian for anxiety. RCTs and systematic reviews provide little evidence that homeopathic medicines are effective for any specific condition. The key ingredient can be extremely diluted, so the principle of action does not appear to be science-based. Even when the main ingredient is highly diluted, there may be other active ingredients in the mixture, including alcohol and metals, that can cause side effects and drug interactions.

Table 63.1. Examples Of Natural Products Marketed To Consumers For Treatment Of Mental Disorders

Product	Example Of Use	Evidence Of Effectiveness	Cautions
Omega-3 fatty acids (found in fatty fish, flax, and other dietary sources)	Depression	May have benefit as an adjunct to standard pharmacologic therapy for depression	May interact with anticoagulants
SAMe (chemical found naturally in the body)	Depression	May have benefit as an adjunct to standard pharmacologic therapy for depression	Close medical supervision is advised for patients with bipolar disorder or on tricyclic antidepressants.
Kava (*Piper methysticum*, plant)	Anxiety	May have anxiolytic effect	Safety risks outweigh benefits. Adversely interacts with several classes of drugs, including some sedatives, benzodiazepines, and monoamine oxidase inhibitors (MAOIs). Has been linked to severe liver damage. Should not be taken with alcohol because of risk of excessive sedation and harm to the liver.
St. John's wort (*Hypericum perforatum*, herb)	Depression	Some evidence exists to support use for treating mild to moderate depression in adults	Active compounds in St. John's wort interact with other medications to render them less effective and potentially cause serious side effects. Such herb–drug interactions have been documented for MAOIs and selective serotonin reuptake inhibitors, used to treat depression. Interactions have also been documented for medications to treat other conditions, including HIV/AIDS, Parkinson disease, and cancer. St. John's wort can also interfere with the efficacy of oral contraceptives, anticonvulsants, immunosuppressants used with transplantation, anticoagulants, and other types of medications. Products made from St. John's wort vary considerably in the quantity and quality of their active compounds, leading to variability in interactive and other side effects.

What Can Complementary And Alternative Medicine (CAM) Do For Anxiety?

Anxiety has now surpassed depression as the most common mental health diagnosis among college students," even though depression is also increasing among young people. In fact, "more than half of students visiting campus clinics cite anxiety as a health concern," according to a recent study of more than 100,000 students nationwide by the Center for Collegiate Mental Health (CCMH) at Penn State.

A yearly survey conducted by the American College Health Association found that "nearly one in six college students has been diagnosed with or treated for anxiety within the last 12 months."

Unlike the relatively mild, brief anxiety caused by a specific event (such as speaking in public or a first date), severe anxiety that lasts at least six months is generally considered to be a problem that might benefit from evaluation and treatment, according to the National Institutes of Health's (NIH) National Institute for Mental Health (NIMH).

Each anxiety disorder has different symptoms, but all the symptoms cluster around excessive, irrational fear and dread. Anxiety disorders commonly occur along with other mental or physical illnesses, including alcohol or substance abuse, which may mask anxiety symptoms or make them worse.

Research studies funded by the NIH's National Center for Complementary and Integrative Health (NCCIH) have investigated several natural products and mind and body practices for anxiety. As with any treatment, it is important to consider safety before using complementary health products and practices. Safety depends on the specific therapy, and each complementary product or practice should be considered on its own.

Mind and body practices such as meditation and yoga, for example, are generally considered to be safe in healthy people when practiced appropriately. Natural products such as herbal medicines or botanicals are often sold as dietary supplements and are readily available to consumers; however, there is a lot we don't know about the safety of many of these products, in part because a manufacturer does not have to prove the safety and effectiveness of a dietary supplement before it is available to the public.

Two of the main safety concerns for dietary supplements are:

- The possibilities of drug interactions—for example, research has shown that St. John's wort interacts with drugs, such as antidepressants, in ways that can interfere with their intended effects.

- The possibilities of product contamination—supplements have been found to contain hidden prescription drugs or other compounds, particularly in dietary supplements marketed for weight loss, sexual health, including erectile dysfunction, and athletic performance or body-building.

Chapter 64

CAM For Attention Deficit Hyperactivity Disorder (ADHD)

People with attention deficit hyperactivity disorder (ADHD) may have trouble paying attention or controlling impulsive behavior, and they may be overly active. Difficulty paying attention is the main problem for some people, hyperactivity and impulsiveness for others. Surveys estimate that as many as 9 percent of American children have ADHD. Conventional treatment for ADHD includes medication, behavior therapy, or a combination of both. Stimulant medication (the most commonly used type of medication) has been shown to be helpful for at least 70 percent of children with ADHD.

Treating ADHD With CAM: What The Science Says

Although conventional treatment has been proven helpful for ADHD symptoms in children and adolescents, complementary approaches have not. Complementary health approaches studied for ADHD include the following:

- **Dietary supplements**
    - The possibility that omega-3 fatty acids could be helpful for ADHD is being investigated, but the evidence is inconclusive.
    - Correcting deficiencies in the minerals zinc, iron, or magnesium may improve ADHD symptoms, but this does not mean that supplements of these minerals would

About This Chapter: Text in this chapter begins with excerpts from "Attention-Deficit Hyperactivity Disorder At A Glance," National Center for Complementary and Integrative Health (NCCIH), September 24, 2017; Text under the heading "Seven Things To Know About Complementary Health Approaches For ADHD" is excerpted from "7 Things To Know About Complementary Health Approaches For ADHD," National Center for Complementary and Integrative Health (NCCIH), September 24, 2015.

be helpful for people with ADHD who are not deficient, and all three minerals can be toxic if taken in excessive amounts.

- Melatonin has not been shown to relieve ADHD symptoms, but it may help children with ADHD who have sleep problems to fall asleep sooner.
- Research on L-carnitine/acetyl-L-carnitine and various herbs, such as St. John's wort, French maritime pine bark extract (also known as Pycnogenol), and *Ginkgo biloba*, has not demonstrated that these supplements are helpful for ADHD.

Omega-3 fatty acids (omega-3s) are a group of polyunsaturated fatty acids that are important for a number of functions in the body. Some types of omega-3s are found in foods such as fatty fish and shellfish. Another type is found in some vegetable oils.

(Source: "Omega-3 Supplements: In Depth," National Center for Complementary and Integrative Health (NCCIH).)

- **Special diets.** Despite much research, the role of foods and food ingredients (such as color additives) in ADHD remains controversial. Some evidence suggests that only a small number of people with ADHD are affected by substances in food, and that different individuals may react to different foods or food components.
- **Neurofeedback.** Some research has suggested that neurofeedback, a technique in which people are trained to alter their brain wave patterns, may improve ADHD symptoms, but several small studies that compared neurofeedback with a simulated (sham) version of the procedure did not find differences between the two treatments.
- **Other complementary health approaches.** An assessment of research on homeopathy concluded that there is no evidence that it is helpful for ADHD symptoms. Several mind and body practices, including acupuncture, chiropractic care, massage therapy, meditation, and yoga, have been studied for ADHD. However, the amount of evidence on each of these practices is small, and no conclusions can be reached about whether they are helpful.

Side Effects And Risks

- Dietary supplements may have side effects and may interact with drugs. In particular, St. John's wort can speed up the process by which the body breaks down many drugs, thus making the drugs less effective. Zinc, iron, and magnesium can all be toxic in high doses.

- If you're interested in trying a special diet, consult your healthcare provider and consider getting guidance from a registered dietitian. Planning, evaluating, and following special diets can be challenging, and it is important to ensure that the diet meets nutritional needs.
- If you're considering using any of the approaches discussed here for ADHD, discuss this decision with your healthcare provider.

Seven Things To Know About Complementary Health Approaches For ADHD

Here are seven things you should know if you are considering a complementary health approach for ADHD:

1. Researchers are studying whether omega-3 fatty acids could be helpful for ADHD, but current evidence is inconclusive.
2. Melatonin has not been shown to relieve ADHD symptoms, but it may help children with ADHD who have sleep problems to fall asleep sooner.
3. Research on other dietary supplements, including L-carnitine, St. John's wort, French maritime pine bark extract (also known as Pycnogenol), and *ginkgo biloba*, has not demonstrated that these supplements are helpful for ADHD. Dietary supplements may have side effects and may interact with drugs. In particular, St. John's wort can speed up the process by which the body breaks down many drugs, thus making the drugs less effective.
4. Several mind and body practices, such as acupuncture, massage therapy, and meditation have been studied for ADHD, but the amount of evidence on each of these practices is small, and no conclusions can be reached about whether they are beneficial.
5. Short-term aerobic exercise, including yoga, has shown beneficial effects on symptoms of ADHD such as attention, hyperactivity, and impulsivity.
6. Some research has suggested that neurofeedback, a technique in which people are trained to alter their brain wave patterns, may improve ADHD symptoms, but several small studies that compared neurofeedback to a control procedure did not find differences between the two treatments.
7. If you're considering using any of these complementary health approaches, or others, for ADHD, talk with your healthcare provider.

Chapter 65

Complementary Health Approaches For Seasonal Affective Disorder (SAD)

Seasonal affective disorder (SAD), a type of depression that comes and goes with the seasons, typically starts in the late fall and early winter and goes away during the spring and summer. Depressive episodes linked to the summer can occur, but are much less common than winter episodes of SAD.

Prevalence Of Seasonal Affective Disorder

SAD is more common in women, young people, and those who live far from the equator. You are also more likely to have SAD if you or your family members have depression.

(Source: "Seasonal Affective Disorder," MedlinePlus, National Institutes of Health (NIH).)

To be diagnosed with SAD, people must meet full criteria for major depression coinciding with specific seasons for at least 2 years. Some of the symptoms of the winter pattern of SAD include having low energy, overeating, craving carbohydrates, and social withdrawal. Light therapy has become a standard treatment of SAD, and antidepressants have also been shown to improve SAD symptoms.

Some people turn to complementary health approaches to prevent SAD, including St. John's wort, melatonin, and vitamin D. This chapter provides the summary of current research for these modalities.

About This Chapter: This chapter includes text excerpted from "Complementary Health Approaches For Seasonal Affective Disorder," National Center for Complementary and Integrative Health (NCCIH), December 2017.

Frequency

SAD occurs in 0.5–3 percent of individuals in the general population; it affects 10–20 percent of people with major depressive disorder and about 25 percent of people with bipolar disorder.

Some individuals have a condition known as subsyndromal seasonal affective disorder or seasonality, which is more common than SAD. These individuals have only mild changes in mood that correspond with the changes in seasons.

(Source: "Seasonal Affective Disorder," Genetics Home Reference (GHR), National Institutes of Health (NIH).)

SAD: What The Science Says

Light Therapy

There is some evidence that light therapy may be useful as a preventive treatment for people with a history of SAD. The idea behind light therapy is to replace the diminished sunshine of the fall and winter months using daily exposure to a light box. Most typically, light boxes filter out the ultraviolet rays and require 20–60 minutes of exposure to 10,000 lux of cool-white fluorescent light, an amount that is about 20 times greater than ordinary indoor lighting.

What Does The Research Show?

- A 2015 Cochrane review of one study involving 46 people concluded that there is limited evidence on light therapy as preventive treatment for patients with a history of SAD. Evidence is limited based on methodological limitations and small sample sizes of studies. The researchers noted that the decision for or against initiating preventive treatment of SAD or using other preventive options should be strongly based on patient preferences.
- A randomized controlled trial of 98 participants examined the effect of light therapy and exercise on depressive symptoms, and found that both treatments, even in combination, seem to be well tolerated and effective on symptoms.
- A randomized controlled trial of 57 participants with SAD found that symptom scores decreased by more than 40 percent after exposure to 4 weeks of bright white or dim red light.

Safety

- Ultraviolet lights should be avoided because of the increased risk of skin cancer.
- People should avoid staring directly into the light to avoid possible retinal injury.
- Side effects are typically mild, and include vision issues such as blurry vision, photophobia, or headache.
- Light therapy may induce mania in patients with unrecognized or undertreated bipolar disorder.

Cognitive Behavioral Therapy (CBT)

There is some evidence that cognitive behavioral therapy (CBT)—SAD can be effective in reducing the recurrence and remissions of SAD and has been shown to be sustained at least between a first and second winter season.

CBT is type of psychotherapy that is effective for SAD. Traditional CBT has been adapted for use with SAD (CBT-SAD). CBT relies on basic techniques of CBT such as identifying negative thoughts and replacing them with more positive thoughts along with a technique called behavioral activation. Behavioral activation seeks to help the person identify activities that are engaging and pleasurable, whether indoors or outdoors, to improve coping with winter.

What Does The Research Show?

A 2016 randomized head-to-head trial of 177 participants found that CBT was superior to light therapy two winters following acute treatment, suggesting greater durability for CBT.

Safety

CBT is generally considered safe for most people.

St. John's Wort

There is limited evidence that St. John's wort may improve some symptoms of SAD; however, the studies have been small.

What Does The Research Show?

- A study of 20 participants who received St. John's wort combined with either bright light or dim light therapy found significant reductions in depressive symptoms in both groups, but no significant difference between the two groups.

- A study of 168 participants with SAD examined the effects of St. John's wort on depressive symptoms and compared results to St. John's wort plus light therapy. Improvement in symptoms were seen in both groups, with no significant differences between them.

Safety

- St. John's wort can weaken the effects of many medicines, including antidepressants, contraceptives, cyclosporine, digoxin, indinavir, irinotecan, and anticoagulants.
- Taking St. John's wort with certain antidepressants or other drugs that affect serotonin may lead to increased serotonin-related side effects, which may be potentially serious.
- St. John's wort may cause increased sensitivity to sunlight. Other side effects can include anxiety, dry mouth, dizziness, gastrointestinal symptoms, fatigue, headache, or sexual dysfunction.

Melatonin

There is some limited evidence (small trials involving few patients) that suggests melatonin improves sleep in some patients with SAD.

What Does The Research Show?

- A Cochrane review found no available methodologically sound evidence indicating that melatonin is or is not an effective intervention for prevention of SAD and improvement of patient-centered outcomes among adults with a history of SAD.
- A controlled study conducted in Europe in 58 participants with SAD or weather-associated mood changes found significant improvements in quality of sleep and vitality in the SAD group; however, melatonin was ineffective in the weather-associated mood group.

Safety

- Melatonin appears to be safe when used short term, but the lack of long-term studies means researchers don't know if it's safe for extended use.
- Side effects of melatonin are uncommon but can include drowsiness, headache, dizziness, or nausea. There have been no reports of significant side effects of melatonin in children.

Vitamin D

At present, vitamin D supplementation by itself is not considered an effective SAD treatment. Low blood levels of vitamin D are often found in people with SAD; however, the evidence for its use has been mixed. Although some studies suggest vitamin D supplementation may be as effective as light therapy, others found vitamin D had no effect.

What Does The Research Show?

- A randomized controlled trial of 34 healthcare professionals failed to demonstrate an effect of vitamin D on SAD symptoms, but the study authors noted that the findings may be limited by confounders.
- A randomized trial of 2,117 women found that daily supplementation of vitamin D did not lead to an improvement in mental health scores.
- A study of 15 participants compared vitamin D and broad spectrum phototherapy in the treatment of SAD. Participants receiving vitamin D improved in all outcome measures, while the phototherapy group had no significant change in depression scale measures.

Safety

- High doses of vitamin D may cause fatigue, abdominal cramps, nausea, vomiting, renal damage, and other adverse effects.

Chapter 66

Skin Conditions And Complementary Health Approaches

Research has shown that people with skin conditions often turn to complementary health approaches, particularly vitamin, mineral, and herbal supplements. In spite of interest in complementary approaches, there have been only a few studies on complementary health approaches for skin conditions, and those that have been conducted have often had methodological problems. This chapter provides a summary of the available evidence about complementary health approaches for skin conditions, including atopic dermatitis, psoriasis, acne, impetigo, and rosacea.

Skin Facts

Skin is actually the body's largest organ. It helps regulate internal temperature, allows the body to retain fluids (preventing dehydration), and keeps harmful microbes out. Skin diseases are very common, and affect as many as one in three Americans at any given time.

(Source: "Skin Conditions At A Glance," National Center for Complementary and Integrative Health (NCCIH).)

About This Chapter: This chapter includes text excerpted from "Skin Conditions And Complementary Health Approaches," National Center for Complementary and Integrative Health (NCCIH), August 2016.

What The Science Says

Atopic Dermatitis

The Evidence Base

The evidence base on efficacy of complementary health approaches for atopic dermatitis consists of several randomized controlled trials on a variety of modalities and clinical practice guidelines from the American Academy of Dermatology (AAD).

Mind And Body Practices

There is some limited evidence that relaxation techniques may help improve symptoms of atopic dermatitis, particularly in the pediatric population, although most clinical studies are not methodologically rigorous. There is currently no evidence that acupuncture has any beneficial effects in the management of atopic dermatitis in adults or children.

Efficacy

- **Acupuncture.** A systematic review of acupuncture found no eligible studies to include in the review, although there were two studies that evaluated the antipruritic effects of acupuncture and one study that evaluated the effects of acupuncture on IgE-mediated allergy, a major characteristic of atopic dermatitis. The reviewers concluded that there is currently no evidence of the effects of acupuncture in the management of atopic dermatitis.
- **Relaxation Techniques.** A small 2012 study of 25 patients with atopic dermatitis concluded that progressive muscle relaxation may be a useful adjunctive modality for the management of atopic dermatitis through the reduction of anxiety.

Safety

- Acupuncture appears to be safe when performed by appropriately trained practitioners, but a research review concluded that unwanted side effects can occur when acupuncture is done by poorly trained practitioners.
- Relaxation techniques are generally considered safe for healthy people, including children. However, there have been rare reports that certain relaxation techniques might cause or worsen symptoms in people with epilepsy or certain psychiatric conditions, or with a history of abuse or trauma.

Natural Products

According to the AAD's clinical practice guidelines for the treatment of atopic dermatitis, there is inconsistent to no evidence to recommend the use of fish oils, evening primrose oil, borage oil, multivitamin supplements, zinc, vitamin D, vitamin E, and vitamins B12 and B6 for the treatment of atopic dermatitis. Further, the guidelines state that the use of probiotics/prebiotics for the treatment of patients with established atopic dermatitis is not recommended because of inconsistent evidence.

Efficacy

- **Dietary Supplements (Oral).** A Cochrane review of 11 randomized controlled trials of dietary supplements (e.g., fish oil, vitamin D and vitamin E, vitamin B6, sea buckhorn oil, hempseed oil, sunflower oil, docosahexaenoic acid (DHA), selenium, and zinc sulfate) for atopic eczema found no convincing evidence of benefit for dietary supplements in atopic eczema. The AAD's *Clinical Practice Guidelines* for the treatment of atopic dermatitis states that "there is inconsistent to no evidence to recommend the use of fish oils, evening primrose oil, borage oil, multivitamin supplements, zinc, vitamin D, vitamin E, and vitamins B12 and B6 for the treatment of atopic dermatitis."
- **Probiotics (Oral).** The AAD's *Clinical Practice Guidelines* for treatment of atopic dermatitis state that "the use of probiotics/prebiotics for the treatment of patients with established atopic dermatitis is not recommended because of inconsistent evidence.
    - There are conflicting data on the efficacy of probiotics for atopic dermatitis in children; overall, evidence suggests that probiotics may be effective for some, but not all, children with atopic dermatitis.
    - A systematic review of 21 randomized controlled trials involving 6,859 participants, which included infants or mothers who were either pregnant or breastfeeding, investigated whether nutrient supplementation with probiotics, prebiotics, formula, or fatty acids prevents the development of atopic dermatitis or reduces the severity of the condition in newborns to children under 3 years of age. Data showed that certain types of nutrient supplementation may be an effective method in preventing atopic dermatitis or decreasing its severity. The best evidence, the reviewers found, lies with probiotics supplementation in mothers and infants in preventing the development and reducing the severity of atopic dermatitis.

  - A Cochrane review of 12 trials found that probiotics do not reduce eczema symptoms such as itching, nor do they change the overall severity of eczema judged by their patients or their doctors.

- **Primrose Oil and Borage Oil (Oral).** A Cochrane review of 27 randomized controlled trials involving a total of 1,596 participants found that evening primrose oil and borage oil taken orally had no clinical benefit for the treatment of atopic eczema.

- **Chinese Herbal Medicine (Oral and Topical).** Another Cochrane review of 28 randomized controlled trials involving a total of 2,306 participants found no conclusive evidence that oral or topical Chinese herbal medicine could reduce the severity of atopic eczema in children or adolescents. A systematic review and meta-analysis of 10 studies involving 1,058 participants found no conclusive evidence demonstrating that topics Chinese herbal medicine for atopic eczema was superior to other control interventions.

Safety

- Patients considering the use of Chinese herbal medicine, especially for children, should use caution as they can be potentially hazardous. A review noted that these medications are easily accessed and not monitored by the U.S. Food and Drug Administration (FDA), and that some topical Chinese herbal medicines have been found to include high concentrations of dexamethasone.

Psoriasis

There is some evidence that fish oil, Dead Sea climatotherapy, and the topical herbs *Mahonia aquifolium* and indigo naturalis may be beneficial for the treatment of psoriasis.

The Evidence Base

The evidence base on efficacy of complementary health approaches for psoriasis consists of several small randomized controlled trials.

Efficacy

- **Traditional Chinese medicine (Oral).** There is some evidence that has shown that the combination of traditional Chinese medicine taken orally with conventional treatments for psoriasis is more efficacious than conventional treatment alone.

- **Dietary supplements (Oral).** A review noted that there has been consistent evidence supporting the efficacy of fish oil supplementation in patients with psoriasis; however, there is conflicting evidence for vitamin D, B12, and selenium supplementation.
- **Herbal medicine (Topical).** A review of complementary health approaches for psoriasis stated that the topical herbal therapies that have the most evidence for efficacy are *Mahonia aquifolium* and indigo naturalis, while there is a smaller amount of evidence for aloe vera, neem, and extracts of sweet whey. A systematic review and meta-analysis of plant extracts for the topical management of psoriasis concluded that there is limited but consistent clinical trial evidence for the efficacy of extracts of *Mahonia aquifolium* and indigo naturalis in plaque psoriasis when compared with the vehicle creams; however, the magnitude and duration of the effects are not assessable based on currently available evidence.

Aloe vera's use can be traced back 6,000 years to early Egypt, where the plant was depicted on stone carvings. Known as the "plant of immortality," aloe was presented as a funeral gift to pharaohs. Two substances from aloe vera, the clear gel and the yellow latex, are used in health products today. Aloe gel is primarily used topically (applied to the skin) as a remedy for skin conditions such as burns, frostbite, psoriasis, and cold sores.

(Source: "Aloe Vera," National Center for Complementary and Integrative Health (NCCIH).)

- **Vitamin D (Topical).** A Cochrane review of 177 studies involving a total of 34,808 people found that topical vitamin D products were superior to placebo, and had similar effects to topical corticosteroids when applied to the body. However, corticosteroids were superior to vitamin D for scalp psoriasis. Treatment that combined topical vitamin D with a corticosteroid was more effective than topical vitamin D alone and more effective than the topical corticosteroid alone.
- **Climatotherapy.** There is evidence from controlled trials that Dead Sea climatotherapy can improve psoriasis and induce lasting remissions; however, research on other locations of climatotherapy have provided little evidence.
- **Light Therapy.** Findings from a randomized controlled trial of 21 patients with plaque psoriasis suggest that moderate to severe plaque psoriasis should show a therapeutic response to orally administered *Curcuma longa* extract if activated with visible light phototherapy. A randomized controlled trial of 47 patients with mild psoriasis vulgaris evaluated the safety and efficacy of long-term ultraviolet (UV)-free blue light treatment and

found that participants receiving blue light treatment had a significant improvement compared to the control.

Safety

- Some Chinese herbal medicines have been shown to be contaminated with heavy metals or corticosteroids. Other safety concerns include systemic toxicity or contact dermatitis from herbal supplements.
- UV light exposure increases the risk of for both melanoma and nonmelanoma skin cancers, so the benefits of climatotherapy should be carefully weighed against the risks for each patient.
- Vitamin D products may cause "local adverse events," such as skin irritation and burning.

Acne

According to the AAD's *Clinical Practice Guidelines* for the treatment of acne, there are very limited data regarding the safety and efficacy of herbal and other complementary therapies to recommend their use.

The Evidence Base

- The evidence base on efficacy of complementary health approaches for acne consists of a few randomized controlled trials and clinical practice guidelines issued by the AAD.

Efficacy

- **Tea tree oil, bee venom (Topical).** A Cochrane review of 35 randomized controlled trials involving 3,227 participants concluded that there is some low-quality evidence from single trials that topical tea tree oil and bee venom may reduce total skin lesions in acne, but there is a lack of evidence from the review to support the use of other complementary health approaches, such as herbal medicine, acupuncture, or wet-cupping therapy. Another review of seven studies concluded that topical use of tea tree oil is an appropriate option for treating mild-to-moderate acne.
- **Barberry extract (Oral).** Other herbal agents, such as oral barberry extract, showed some beneficial effects in a randomized controlled trial of 49 adolescents with moderate to severe acne.

- **Biofeedback.** There is weak evidence of the potential benefit of biofeedback-assisted relaxation and cognitive imagery in people with acne. A randomized controlled trial of 30 patients with acne evaluated the efficacy of biofeedback relaxation and cognitive imagery over 6 weeks and found that the treatment group had a significant reduction in acne severity compared to the control groups.

Safety

In a study, oral aqueous extract of barberry was well tolerated, and no notable complications or side effects were reported.

Tea tree oil contains varying amounts of 1,8–cineole, a skin irritant. Products with high amounts of this compound may cause skin irritation or contact dermatitis in some individuals. Oxidized tea tree oil may trigger allergies more than fresh tea tree oil.

Tea tree oil should not be swallowed. Poisonings, mainly in children, have caused drowsiness, disorientation, rash, and ataxia. Topical use of diluted tea tree oil is generally considered safe for most adolescents. Pruritus, burning, stinging, scaling, itch, redness, and dryness have been reported.

There is a potential for adverse effects from herbal medicines. Patients considering the use of Chinese herbal medicine, especially for children, should use caution as they can be potentially hazardous. A review noted that these medications are easily accessed and not monitored by the FDA, and that some topical Chinese herbal medicines have been found to include high concentrations of dexamethasone.

Impetigo

There is insufficient evidence to either recommend or dismiss herbal treatments for impetigo, including tea tree oil, garlic, coconut oils, tea effusions, and Manuka honey.

The evidence base on efficacy of herbal extracts for impetigo consists of only a few controlled clinical trials, most of which are not methodologically rigorous.

Efficacy

Herbal medicine (Oral and topical). A review of seven randomized and nonrandomized studies examining both oral and topical herbal medicines for the treatment of bacterial infections, including impetigo, found some positive results reported for a topical ointment containing tea leaf extract. However, the reviewers concluded that the clinical efficacy of none of the herbal medicines has so far been demonstrated.

Safety

There is a lack of safety data on herbal medicines for the treatment of impetigo. Patients should be encouraged to maintain proper wound care and hand washing and avoid contact with others as the infection can spread.

Rosacea

Although some natural products have shown promise for improving symptoms of rosacea, there is insufficient evidence to support the use of many of these products for rosacea.

The Evidence Base

The evidence base on efficacy of natural products for rosacea consists of several clinical studies, but most of these studies are not methodologically rigorous.

Efficacy

- **Plant extracts (Oral and topical).** A systematic review of phytochemical and botanical therapies for rosacea found that several botanical therapies may be promising for rosacea symptoms, with several plant extracts and phytochemicals improving facial erythema and papule/pustule counts caused by rosacea. However, many of the studies included in the review were not methodologically rigorous.
- **Azelaic acid (Topical).** A review of natural products had similar findings, but noted that based on two randomized trials, topical azelaic acid—a naturally occurring 9-carbon acid found in whole grain cereals and animal products—may provide some benefit for symptoms of rosacea.

Safety

The systematic review of various phytochemical and botanical therapies found mild adverse reactions, such as transient burning or pruritus, and noted that several botanicals commonly used for rosacea have not been studied clinically and these may have more significant side effect profiles.

A review of two studies found azelaic acid to be generally safe, with mild and transient local adverse reactions, and no difference between azelaic acid and placebo.

Part Nine
If You Need More Information

Chapter 67

Clinical Trials And CAM

Clinical trials are an important part of medical research. They help scientists find better ways to prevent, detect, and treat diseases and medical conditions. This chapter provides an introduction to clinical trials in general and also to trials involving complementary and alternative medicine (CAM).

Key Points

- Clinical trials are research studies in which the safety and efficacy of treatments and therapies are tested in people. Clinical trials are essential for determining which treatments work, which do not, and why.
- There are clinical trials for healthy people (for example, to prevent disease) and trials for many different types and stages of diseases and conditions.
- Participating in a clinical trial can have benefits and risks; the Federal Government requires that participants in federally funded clinical trials are protected and closely monitored. All known risks must be disclosed to participants before they enter a study.
- If you are interested in taking part in a clinical trial, talk with your healthcare provider. Also, be sure that you understand the information contained in the consent form, have had all of your questions answered, and have discussed the decision with family, friends, or other people you trust.

About This Chapter: This chapter includes text excerpted from "Clinical Trials And CAM," National Center for Complementary and Integrative Health (NCCIH), August 2010. Reviewed January 2018.

About CAM

CAM is a group of diverse medical and healthcare systems, practices, and products that are not generally considered part of conventional medicine. Complementary medicine is used together with conventional medicine, and alternative medicine is used in place of conventional medicine.

Overview Of Clinical Trials

A clinical trial is a research study in which a treatment or therapy is tested in people to see whether it is safe and effective. Clinical trials also help researchers learn which treatments are more effective than others. The information gained from clinical trials helps to improve medical care and contributes to the understanding of diseases and conditions (for example, how a disease progresses or how it affects different systems in the body).

Clinical trials are also called medical research, research studies, or clinical studies. Each trial follows a protocol, which is a written, detailed plan that explains why the study is needed, what it is intended to do, and how it will be conducted. The protocol is written by the trial's principal investigator (the person in charge of the trial).

Types Of Clinical Trials

Clinical trials are used to study many aspects of healthcare:

- **Treatment trials** test treatments for a specific disease or condition.
- **Prevention trials** study ways to reduce the chance that people who are healthy, but possibly at risk for a disease, will develop the disease.
- **Early detection or screening trials** study new ways of finding diseases or conditions before they produce signs or symptoms.
- **Diagnostic trials** test new ways to identify, more accurately and earlier, whether people have diseases and conditions.
- Supportive care trials, also called **quality-of-life trials**, study ways of making patients more comfortable and giving them a better quality of life.

There is a common misunderstanding that clinical trials are a last resort for those who have a disease and have tried all other treatment options. However, there are trials for healthy people (for example, to study disease prevention) and for all different types and stages of diseases.

Clinical Trial Phases

Because a clinical trial tests treatments in people, there needs to be some evidence before the clinical trial starts that the therapy is likely to work. This evidence can come either from previous laboratory research studies or from reports on the therapy's use by people.

Clinical trials take place in phases. In Phase I trials, researchers test the treatment in a small group of people, focusing on safety, adverse effects, and sometimes dosage and schedule of administration. In Phase II trials, the treatment is given to a larger number of people to determine potential usefulness and to further evaluate its safety and adverse effects. This phase can last several years. In Phase III trials, the treatment is usually given to several hundred or more people to confirm its efficacy and more fully define any adverse effects. Phase III trials often compare the treatment under study with standard treatments.

In each phase, different research questions are answered:

- **Phase I:** What is the safe dose? How does the treatment affect the human body? How should the treatment be given?
- **Phase II:** Does the therapy cause any adverse effects? Are the adverse effects tolerable? Is there evidence that the therapy is useful in treating the disease or condition?
- **Phase III:** Is the treatment better than, the same as, or worse than placebo or a standard (and widely accepted) treatment or approach?

Common Elements Of Clinical Trials

Trials can be randomized. In a randomized trial, each participant is assigned by chance—through a computer or a table of random numbers—to either an investigational group or a control group. Randomization is used in all Phase III studies and in some Phase II studies. It helps ensure that the study results are attributable to the treatment and not to unrelated factors that might bias the outcome or the interpretation of the results.

Each participant has an equal chance of being assigned to any group. Some complex trials include several groups.

Trials are often double blind. This means that neither the researchers nor the participants know who has been assigned to which group. Blinding is another way to help minimize the chance of bias influencing the trial results. The information is kept on file at a central office so the research team can find out who was assigned the active treatment if they need to know.

Researchers design clinical trials to have one or more endpoints. An endpoint is a measure that determines whether the treatment under study has an important effect. An example of an endpoint is whether a person's pain improves following acupuncture treatment.

About Placebos

A placebo is an inactive treatment designed to resemble the treatment being studied. An example of a placebo is a pill containing sugar instead of the drug being studied. By giving one group of participants a placebo and the other group the active treatment, the researchers can compare how the two groups respond. This gives the researchers a truer picture of the active treatment's effects.

Another type of placebo, called a "sham," is used when the treatment under study is a procedure (e.g., acupuncture), not a drug or other substance. A sham procedure is designed to simulate the active treatment but does not have any active treatment qualities. For example, in a clinical trial of acupuncture, the sham procedure might consist of placing acupuncture needles in areas of the body that are not expected to have any therapeutic response.

Placebos are necessary because many factors other than the treatment being studied can influence either the course of an illness or the response of a patient to treatment. For example, many illnesses or symptoms resolve on their own, and interactions with the provider or a patient's expectations about the treatment may influence the patient's response. These and other factors are part of what is known as the "placebo effect," which researchers try to separate from the effects of the treatment they are studying.

About Participants

Each clinical trial is unique in its eligibility criteria—i.e., rules for who can participate. The purpose of the criteria is to identify appropriate participants, based on what is being studied and the questions the researchers hope to answer. Examples of criteria include type or severity of disease, presence of other illnesses, and history of prior treatment.

As much as possible, clinical trials include people of various ages and ethnic groups and both genders so the results can apply to the general population. Sometimes, because of what is being studied, it makes sense for a trial to be limited to a particular group, such as women or older people. Eligibility criteria are also intended to make the trial as safe as possible for participants. For example, it might not be safe for someone with a serious illness to participate if they would have to stop taking their regular medicine to do so. The criteria are never used to exclude someone for reasons not related to the study itself.

NIH Protections For Study Participants: Historical Context

The National Institutes of Health (NIH) has established policies and procedures to protect people involved in research studies. The foundation of the NIH protections is The Belmont Report—Ethical Principles and Guidelines for the Protection of Human Subjects. Published in 1979, the Belmont Report provides the philosophical basis for current Federal laws governing research that involves people. It established three fundamental ethical principles for such research: respect for persons, beneficence (maximizing benefits and minimizing harms), and justice (treating subjects fairly). Another document in the history of protections for research participants is The Declaration of Helsinki: Recommendations Guiding Medical Doctors in Biomedical Research Involving Human Subjects, issued in 1964 by the World Medical Association. The Declaration of Helsinki broadened concepts initially set forth after World War II in The Nuremberg Code, which named 10 conditions that must be met to justify research involving people. The two most important conditions were the need for voluntary informed consent of participants and a scientifically valid research design that could produce fruitful results for the good of society.

Protections For Participants

The Federal Government requires many protections for people who participate in federally funded clinical trials. Before a clinical trial can start, the written protocol must be approved and monitored by an institutional review board (IRB)—an independent group of healthcare providers, other experts, and people from the community who make sure that the study is set up and run safely and fairly. IRBs also review and approve the consent documents that people must sign in order to participate in a clinical trial. An IRB can stop a clinical trial if the researcher is not following the protocol or if the trial appears to be causing unexpected harm to the participants. An IRB can also stop a clinical trial if the evidence is clear that the new intervention is effective so that it can be made widely available as soon as possible.

At NIH, clinical trials also require additional data and safety monitoring. Some clinical trials—especially Phase III clinical trials, which often involve many institutions—use a Data Safety Monitoring Board (DSMB). A DSMB is an independent committee made up of statisticians, physicians, and patient advocates (a majority of whom are not connected with the clinical trial) who regularly monitor data from the trial to ensure that the risks of participation are as small as possible. Their priority is patient safety—they can stop a trial if safety concerns arise or if the trial's objectives have been met.

Participants are also protected by a process called informed consent. People who are considering taking part in a clinical trial meet with a member of the research team, who provides key facts about the study, such as:

- Who is sponsoring and conducting the research
- Who has reviewed and approved the study
- What the researchers want to learn
- How the research team will monitor participants' health and safety
- What participants will be required to do during the trial, and for how long
- Possible benefits and risks of participating
- Other treatments that are available for the disease or condition
- How the privacy of participants' medical records will be protected.

Informed Consent Process

When you talk to a member of the research team during the informed consent process, you have a right to have all of your questions answered. If you do not understand an answer you receive, ask again. It can be helpful to make a list of questions and concerns before you talk to the study team.

The staff will also give you a consent form, which explains the study and should be written in straightforward language. Consent forms can be long, and they contain a lot of information that you need to consider carefully. It is a good idea to take the consent form home, so you can think about it and review it with family members or friends. If you are interested in joining a study, it is also very helpful to discuss it with your primary healthcare provider. By signing the form, you are providing your consent to participate in the trial. However, participating in a clinical trial is completely voluntary. You can leave the trial at any time—and for any reason—even after you have signed the consent form.

What Happens During The Trial

What happens depends on the type of trial and the study protocol. However, some activities are similar for all clinical trials:

- The research team will check the participants' health at the beginning of the trial, give specific instructions for participating, and monitor their healthcare fully during the trial.
- Participants may be required to perform some tasks between appointments, such as taking medication according to a schedule, completing logs, or answering questionnaires.

Clinical trials take place in a variety of settings depending on the type of trial and what is being studied. For example, participants in a trial of an herb might follow the protocol at home, while a trial that involves specialized equipment (such as acupuncture) might be carried out in a clinic or other healthcare setting. Other trials may require participants to be in a hospital, clinic, or research center while the therapy is given.

What Happens After The Clinical Trial

The researchers carefully analyze the data from the trial and then consider what their findings mean. If the trial has been completed and the results have medical importance, the researchers share their findings with the medical community and the public. The results are usually reported in a peer-reviewed medical journal ("peer-reviewed" means that the report is reviewed before publication by a group of experts in the same field) and/or discussed at scientific meetings. The media may also cover the results of the study. The research team also will inform the participants about the study results soon after the study is completed and all its data are analyzed. Participants should ask the study team when they expect to know the results.

A treatment that has been found to be safe and effective in a carefully conducted clinical trial may become a new standard practice.

CAM Clinical Trials

Although many CAM treatments have been in use for a long time (sometimes for centuries), there may be less scientific knowledge available about them than for conventional medical approaches. Without scientific evidence, people already using CAM treatments may be at risk—for example, for serious effects from taking the wrong dose, using the treatment in the wrong way, or using it with other medications that may cause a dangerous interaction. Or, the treatment may be ineffective. Researchers, including many supported by National Center for Complementary and Integrative Health (NCCIH), are studying CAM treatments in clinical trials to find answers to questions such as:

- Does it work?
- If so, how does it work?
- For which diseases and conditions does it work?
- What dose is safe?
- What dose is effective for a specific disease or condition?
- What are the adverse effects?

- How should it be given?
- Are there situations in which it might be harmful?
- Can it be used safely with other forms of treatment?
- Is it better than, or a useful option compared with, other treatments that are available?

NCCIH funds studies on a variety of CAM treatments. A few examples include acupuncture; natural products, such as herbs and other dietary supplements; massage; meditation; and chiropractic or osteopathic manipulation. Examples of diseases and conditions for which CAM therapies are studied include cancer, cardiovascular disease, neurological disorders, and osteoarthritis. Some of these studies involve partnerships with other components of NIH. Institutions outside the Federal Government are conducting studies as well.

If You Are Thinking About Participating In A Clinical Trial: Possible Benefits And Risks

Benefits

- You may have the chance to receive expert medical care and have your health closely watched throughout the study.
- Clinical trials can offer an opportunity for excellent treatment or prevention of a disease or condition.
- In some types of trials, you may be among the first to benefit from a new treatment or new knowledge about a current treatment.
- You will help others by helping to advance medical and scientific knowledge.

Risks

- The treatment under study does not always turn out to be better than, or even as good as, standard treatment. The researchers hope that it is, but they need to do the study to find out for certain.
- The treatment may have adverse effects that are unknown to the researchers or different from what they expect.
- If you are in a randomized trial, you may be assigned to a treatment other than the one you hope to receive. You usually will not know what group you are in.
- The treatment under study may not work for everyone.
- Participation may require more tests and more visits or treatments than regular care.
- There may be costs to participate, and these costs may not all be covered by health insurance plans. Be sure to talk with the research team about any costs involved.

Finding CAM Clinical Trials

The NCCIH website contains a listing of NCCIH-funded clinical trials. ClinicalTrials.gov is a database of thousands of clinical studies being sponsored by NIH, other Federal agencies, and the pharmaceutical industry. You can also find out more by contacting the NCCIH Clearinghouse. See "For More Information" below for these and other resources.

For More Information

NCCIH Clearinghouse

The NCCIH Clearinghouse provides information on CAM and NCCIH, including publications and searches of Federal databases of scientific and medical literature. The Clearinghouse does not provide medical advice, treatment recommendations, or referrals to practitioners.

Toll-free in the U.S.: 888-644-6226

TTY (for deaf and hard-of-hearing callers): 866-464-3615

Website: nccih.nih.gov

E-mail: info@nccih.nih.gov

National Institutes of Health (NIH)

NIH—the Nation's medical research agency—includes 27 institutes and centers and is a component of the U.S. Department of Health and Human Services (HHS). It is the primary Federal agency for conducting and supporting basic, clinical, and translational medical research, and it investigates the causes, treatments, and cures for both common and rare diseases.

Website: www.nih.gov

E-mail: nihinfo@od.nih.gov

ClinicalTrials.gov

ClinicalTrials.gov is a database of information on federally and privately supported clinical trials (research studies in people) for a wide range of diseases and conditions. It is sponsored by NIH and the U.S. Food and Drug Administration (FDA).

Website: www.clinicaltrials.gov

PubMed®

A service of the National Library of Medicine (NLM), PubMed® contains publication information and (in most cases) brief summaries of articles from scientific and medical journals. CAM on PubMed®, developed jointly by NCCIH and NLM, is a subset of the PubMed system and focuses on the topic of CAM.

Website: www.ncbi.nlm.nih.gov/sites/entrez

CAM on PubMed®: nccih.nih.gov/research/camonpubmed

Chapter 68

Additional Reading About CAM

Mobile Apps For CAM

Acupuncture HandBook

Acupuncture HandBook is a collection of procedures involving penetration of the skin with needles to stimulate certain points on the body. In its classical form it is a characteristic component of traditional Chinese medicine (TCM), a form of alternative medicine, and one of the oldest healing practices in the world.
Website: play.google.com/store/apps/details?id=com.galakarlabs.acupunturehandbook.AOUJABEPULEZAGRS&hl=en

Alternative Medicine

This app offers information on numerous forms of alternative medicine—likely some you've never even heard of! Whether you're new to the world of alternative and complementary medicine, or a professional practitioner, this app is a useful addition to your mobile library.
Website: play.google.comstore/apps/details?id=andy.almed

Ayurveda Home Remedies & Herbs

Ayurveda Home Remedies & Herbs can help learn to apply time-tested principles to your modern life. You'll find tips and treatments for everything from headaches to yellowing teeth. You can search by symptom or by herb.
Website: play.google.comstore/apps/details?id=com.healthfitness.ayurvedichomeremedies

About This Chapter: The mobile apps listed in this chapter were compiled from several sources deemed reliable. Inclusion does not constitute endorsement, and there is no implication associated with omission. All website information was verified and updated in January 2018.

Breathe Deep

This app is designed to help you learn deep breathing techniques that can help you relax, sleep better, improve your health, and reduce stress. The app contains sessions from 1–15 minutes long, making it a solution for even the busiest practitioners.
Website: itunes.apple.comus/app/breathe-deep-personal-assistant-for-breathing-meditation/id1141679494?mt=8

Breathing Zone

Breathing Zone is a doctor recommended guided breathing exercise. In just 5 minutes you can start to enjoy the deep relaxation and other health benefits of slower therapeutic breathing.
Website: play.google.com/store/apps/details?id=com.breathing.zone&hl=en

Cures A-Z

The Cures A–Z app guides you in treating health issues using the best of the natural and prescription tools available. With hundreds of different health conditions, this powerful tool uses straightforward and easy-to-understand interface to find the best health advice supported by tens of thousands of studies in a matter of seconds.
Website: play.google.com/store/apps/details?id=com.cures.naturalcures&hl=en

Free Hypnosis

This app lets you choose symptoms you'd like to address and in exchange provides hypnotherapy treatments. Though there are in-app purchases, the app comes loaded with over 100 hours of free hypnosis audio.
Websites: itunes.apple.comus/app/free-hypnosis/id438205784?mt=8; play.google.comstore/apps/details?id=com.Hypnosis&hl=en

Handbook of Natural Medicine

Handbook of Natural Medicine is an app version of The Clinician's Handbook of Natural Medicine. In it, you'll find help diagnosing and treating conditions with natural solutions. You can search by keyword or even use your camera to snap a photo of the words you wish to look up.
Website: play.google.comstore/apps/details?id=com.mobisystems.msdict.embedded.wireless.elsevier.naturalmedicine

Healing Hypnosis Meditation

By utilizing the science of psychoneuroimmunology, the healing hypnosis app helps users feel and influence how well we cope and recover from illness and injuries. This app features a powerful hypnosis session designed to help you relax and accelerate the body's natural healing processes.
Website: play.google.com/store/apps/details?id=com.app.healinghypnosis&hl=en

HealthSmart

Healthsmart provides detailed information on health conditions, human anatomy, medical news, and alternative medicine.
Website: play.google.com/store/apps/details?id=com.future.HealthSmart&hl=en

HelloMind

HelloMind is a tool for folks wanting to practice mindfulness and those interested in meditation. Select the behavior or condition you wish to improve, like self-esteem, and the app recommends a relaxation and hypnotherapy treatment for you.
Website: itunes.apple.comus/app/hellomind-meditation-relaxation-and-hypnotherapy/id327538172?mt=8

Herbs Encyclopedia

Herbs Encyclopedia app is a database including a list of herbs and plants, each identified by the symptoms and health concerns it may be useful for. The app also features a list of herbs you shouldn't take—or those that may be harmful if used incorrectly or used at all.
Website: play.google.comstore/apps/details?id=com.e_steps.herbs

Home Remedies+: Natural Cures

Home Remedies+ app identifies home remedies for hundreds of ailments. It also contains remedies for overall wellness, like improving immune health. You can make a list of favorites and even add your own home remedies to the database.
Website: play.google.comstore/apps/details?id=com.hrfy.plus

iTherapy

This app covers everything from acupuncture to Shiatsu, as well as precautions and reasons to do these things in the first place. A good starting point for alternative medicine apps.
Website: itunes.apple.com/us/app/itherapy/id981786230?mt=8

Natural Medicines Database

Natural Medicines Comprehensive Database consists of multiple databases and interactive features including the Effectiveness Checker, Nutrient Depletion Checker, Natural Product/Drug Interaction Checker, Natural Medicines Brand Evidence-based Ratings (NMBER®), as well as accredited continuing medical education modules accredited for physicians, pharmacists, nurse practitioners, physician assistants, and dietitians.
Websites: play.google.com/store/apps/details?id=trc.nmcd; itunes.apple.com/us/app/id512681918?mt=8

The Natural Remedies

This app is a comprehensive but simply designed directory of natural remedies you can find at home or in the wild. It also features vibrant photos of these remedies. You can visually identify herbs found in your backyard and determine how they may be useful in your home healthcare. The tool also includes news from the latest scientific studies on natural health.
Websites: itunes.apple.comus/app/the-natural-remedies/id1081776412; play.google.comstore/apps/details?id=com.kaleidosstudio.natural_remedies

101 Natural Home Remedies Cure

This app is a tool for locating basic home remedy recipes for a variety of symptoms. You'll find solutions for the common cold, high blood pressure, and so much more.
Website: play.google.comstore/apps/details?id=com.xlabz.homeremedies

Optimism

Optimism app allows users to record potential "triggers" or "occurrences" that negatively affect their mental health. By constantly keeping their mood and environment in check, users learn to recognize key triggers and head off bouts of depression or anxiety before they occur. Overall, it functions as a de-stressor promoting mental wellness.
Website: play.google.com/store/apps/details?id=app.consultartecnologia.optimism&hl=en

Sanjivani-Ayurvedic Remedies

Ayurveda or Ayurvedic Medicine is a system of traditional medicine native to Indians and is a form of alternative medicine. This app provides you with some easy cures of most common diseases in real life. One can save money by curing himself using this app.
Website: play.google.com/store/apps/details?id=com.vue.sanjivani&hl=en

SuperBetter

Routinely accomplishing a task doesn't work for everyone, that's why some people seem reluctant to achieve new heights—but not there can be no excuses anymore. The SuperBetter app helps users work toward specific goals such as reducing anxiety, weight loss, or anything under the sun—by allowing you to create your superhero identity and adventure. Stay on top of you game and your life, with SuperBetter.
Website: play.google.com/store/apps/details?id=com.superbetter.paid&hl=en

Internet Resources

Aetna InteliHealth®

Website: www.custom.aetna.com/Inova/intelihealth.shtml

American Heart Association

Healthy Eating Resource
Website: www.recipes.heart.org

Cancer Care
Website: www.cancercare.org

Cancer Clinical Trials Directory
U.S. National Library of Medicine (NLM)
Website: www.clinicaltrials.gov

Centers for Disease Control and Prevention (CDC)
Health Topics A–Z
Website: www.cdc.gov/az

Centerwatch Clinical Trials Listing Service
Website: www.centerwatch.com

Chinese Medicine Sampler
Website: www.chinesemedicinesampler.com

The Cochrane Collaboration
Website: www.cochrane.org

Consumer and Patient Health Information Section (CAPHIS)
(From the Medical Library Association (MLA))
Website: www.mlanet.org/caphis

ConsumerLab.com
Website: www.consumerlab.com

Drug Information
(Over-the-counter and Prescription)
A service of the U.S. National Library of Medicine
Website: www.medlineplus.gov/druginformation.html

Food and Nutrition Information Center (FNIC)—Alternative Medicine
Complementary and Alternative Medicine
Website: www.nal.usda.gov/fnic/complementary-and-alternative-medicine

Health On the Net Foundation
Website: www.hon.ch

Healthfinder
U.S. Department of Health and Human Services (HHS)
Website: www.healthfinder.gov

HealthWorld Online
Website: www.healthy.net

Hepatitis C Choices
(Published by Hepatitis C Caring Ambassadors Program)
Website: www.hepcchallenge.org

Hepatitis C Support Project (HCSP)/HCV Advocate
Website: www.hcvadvocate.org

HerbMed
Website: www.herbmed.org

Jiva Ayurveda
Website: www.jiva.com

Medicinal Herb Garden—University of Washington
Website: www.staff.washington.edu/boerm/uwmhg

MedlinePlus—Complementary and Alternative Therapies Topics
Website: www.medlineplus.gov/complementaryandalternativetherapies.html

Memorial Sloan Kettering (MSK) Cancer Center
Website: www.mskcc.org/cancer-care/diagnosis-treatment/symptom-management/integrative-medicine/herbs

National Cancer Institute (NCI)
Website: www.cancer.gov

National Institutes of Health (NIH)
Website: www.nih.gov

New York Online Access to Health (NOAH)—Complementary and Alternative Medicine
Website: www.noah-health.org

PubMed Dietary Supplement Subset
Website: www.ods.od.nih.gov/Research/PubMed_Dietary_Supplement_Subset.aspx

Quackwatch
Website: www.quackwatch.org

Research Council for Complementary Medicine (RCCM)
Website: www.rccm.org.uk

Savvy Patients
Integrative Medicine Information
Website: www.savvypatients.com

Stanford University Clinical Trials
Website: www.clinicaltrials.stanford.edu

U.S. Department of Health and Human Services and Agriculture
Website: www.hhs.gov/civil-rights/for-individuals/special-topics/national-origin/tri-agency/index.html

U.S. Food and Drug Administration (FDA)
Center for Food Safety and Applied Nutrition
Website: www.fda.gov/AboutFDA/CentersOffices/OfficeofFoods/CFSAN

United States Pharmacopeia
Website: www.usp.org

Utilization Review Accreditation Commission (URAC) Health Website Accreditation
Website: www.urac.org

Vegetarian Starter Kit
From the Physicians Committee for Responsible Medicine (PCRM)
Website: www.pcrm.org/health/diets/vsk

WebMD
Website: www.webmd.com

Magazines, Journals, And Newsletters

Alternative And Complementary Therapies

Alternative and Complementary Therapies is a journal delivering practical and evidence-based research on integrating alternative medical therapies and approaches into private practice or hospital integrative medicine programs. It offers the latest research and top thinking in complementary and alternative medicine (CAM) as it relates to key areas such as the prevention and treatment of chronic illness, mind/body approaches to disease management, and clinical applications of CAM therapies.
Website: www.liebertpub.com/ACT

Alternative Medicine Magazine

Alternative Medicine magazine examines overlooked or dismissed natural approaches to health that are often discarded by modern science and the medical industry. Discussing topics, such as acupuncture, chiropractic medicine, herbal medicine, eastern medicine, and other alternative practices, Alternative Medicine also spotlights conditions and how alternative treatments may work on them. Focused on a natural approach to a healthy lifestyle.
Website: www.alternativemedicine.com

Alternative Therapies In Health And Medicine

Alternative Therapies in Health and Medicine promotes the art and science of integrative medicine and a responsibility to improve public health. It does not endorse any particular system or method but promotes the evaluation and appropriate use of all effective therapeutic approaches. Each issue contains a variety of disciplined inquiry methods, from case reports to original scientific research to systematic reviews.
Website: www.alternative-therapies.com

American Botanical Council (ABC)

American Botanical Council, also known as the Herbal Medicine Institute is passionate about helping people live healthier lives through the responsible use of herbs, medicinal plants. ABC is an independent, nonprofit research, and education organization dedicated to providing accurate and reliable information for consumers, healthcare practitioners, researchers, educators, industry, and the media.
Website: www.abc.herbalgram.org/site/PageServer

BioMed Central (BMC) Complementary And Alternative Medicine

BMC Complementary and Alternative Medicine is an open access journal publishing original peer-reviewed research articles on interventions and resources that complement or replace conventional therapies, with a specific emphasis on research that explores the biological mechanisms of action, as well as their efficacy, safety, costs, patterns of use, and/or implementation.
Website: www.bmccomplementalternmed.biomedcentral.com

Delicious Living

Delicious Living provides online and print recipes for the natural living community, helping us to connect with our local natural products stores and the responsible companies that make healthy living achievable, sustainable, and fun.
Website: www.deliciousliving.com

Direction: A Journal On The Alexander Technique

Direction Journal is the only independent industry journal for the Alexander Technique community worldwide. It provides information and training for Alexander Technique teachers and also for the benefit of their students and to assist them in reaching the wider community.
Website: www.directionjournal.com

Explore: The Journal Of Science And Healing

Explore: The Journal of Science and Healing addresses the scientific principles behind, and applications of, evidence-based healing practices from a wide variety of sources, including conventional, alternative, and cross-cultural medicine. It is an interdisciplinary journal that explores the healing arts, consciousness, spirituality, eco-environmental issues, and basic science as all these fields relate to health.
Website: www.explorejournal.com

Harvard Health Letter

Harvard Health Letter floods you with health news and answers your questions about where to find the best treatment, which food, supplement, or exercise is best for you, and, ultimately, what's the right answer! Each month, the doctors at Harvard Medical School answer questions in the pages of the Harvard Health Letter. Easy-to-read, clear, and concise, Harvard Health Letter is like a monthly conversation with your favorite doctor.
Website: www.health.harvard.edu

Holistic Primary Care

Holisticprimarycare.net provides health-conscious readers and healthcare professionals with a credible source of scientifically-sound information on natural medicine and holistic healthcare. The site is an online extension of Holistic Primary Care-News for Health & Healing, a print publication that reaches approximately 100,000 physicians nationwide.
Website: www.holisticprimarycare.net

Integrative Cancer Therapies

Integrative Cancer Therapies (ICT) is a peer-reviewed quarterly journal focused on a comprehensive model of integrative cancer treatment. This model embraces both conventional healthcare and integrative therapies such as diet, lifestyle, exercise, stress care, and nutritional supplementation.
Website: www.journals.sagepub.comhome/ict

Integrative Medicine: A Clinician's Journal

Integrative Medicine: A Clinician's Journal (IMCJ) provides practitioners with a practical and comprehensive approach to integrating alternative therapies with conventional medicine. The journal is published six times per year under the leadership of Joseph Pizzorno, ND, editor in chief, a co-founder and former president of Bastyr University.
Website: www.imjournal.com

Journal Of Alternative And Complementary Medicine

The Journal of Alternative and Complementary Medicine is a journal providing scientific research for the evaluation and integration of complementary and alternative medicine into mainstream medical practice. The Journal delivers original research that directly impacts patient care therapies, protocols, and strategies, ultimately improving the quality of healing.
Website: www.liebertpub.com/acm

Medical News Today

Medical News Today (MNT) provides concise and accurate information that stands out in the ocean of content that is health on the internet. It is targeted to an educated audience of both healthcare professionals and patients alike. It provides news from evidence-based, peer-reviewed studies, along with accurate, unbiased, and informative content from governmental organizations (e.g., FDA, CDC, NIH, NHS), medical societies, royal colleges, professional associations, patients' groups, pharmaceutical and biotech companies, among others.
Website: www.medicalnewstoday.com

Medscape Today

Medscape is an online global destination for physicians and healthcare professionals worldwide, offering the latest medical news and expert perspectives; essential point-of-care drug and disease information; and relevant professional education and complementary medicine.
Website: www.medscape.com/multispecialty

National Center for Complementary and Integrative Health (NCCIH) Clinical Digest

The NCCIH Clinical Digest is a monthly e-newsletter that summarizes the state of the science on complementary and integrative health practices for a health condition (diabetes, cancer, sleep disorders, etc.)—clinical guidelines, literature searches, continuing medical education, and information for patients.
Website: www.nccih.nih.gov/health/providers/digest

Natural Solutions Magazine

Natural Solutions: Vibrant Health, Balanced Living (formerly Alternative Medicine) guides and inspires people to make conscious choices and helps them to live in a natural lifestyle. It's content reflects the readers' commitment to healthy, natural living. In every issue, it highlights health information pertaining to all aspects of our lives—food, beauty, family, pets, home, and beyond.
Website: www.naturalsolutionsmag.com

Nutrition Action Health Letter

Nutrition Action Health Letter is loaded with practical tips for eating right, cooking healthful recipes, and avoiding food-safety dangers, as well as news of the latest developments in nutrition and health.
Website: www.cspinet.org/nutrition-action-healthletter

Prevention Magazine

Prevention is an American healthy lifestyle magazine based in Pennsylvania, United States. The range of subjects includes food, nutrition, workouts, beauty, and cooking. It's a guide to a healthy lifestyle: Learn how to lower blood pressure, improve gut health, ease seasonal allergies, and sleep better. Pick up tips for treating common health conditions from yeast infections to sciatica to the flu.
Website: www.prevention.com

Qi: The Journal of Traditional Eastern Health & Fitness

Qi-Journal.com helps promote traditional Chinese culture and medicine throughout the world. It's goal is to educate the Western public about the benefits of the ancient Chinese methods of health and fitness.
Website: www.qi-journal.com

Science Daily

Science Daily provides breaking news about the latest scientific discoveries in a user-friendly format—all freely accessible with no subscription fees. With over 200,000 research articles covering science, health, technology, and the environment.
Website: www.sciencedaily.comnews/health_medicine/alternative_medicine

Spirituality & Health

Spirituality & Health covers a broad range of topics under the umbrella of health and spirituality, which can include faith, Eastern philosophy, meditation, and mainstream religion; nutrition, wellness, yoga, and holistic medicine; creativity, the inner life, social justice, and issues of conscience; and public health, the human body, and the environment.
Website: www.spiritualityhealth.com

Townsend Letter: The Examiner Of Alternative Medicine

Townsend Letter, the Examiner of Alternative Medicine, publishes a print magazine about alternative medicine. It is written by researchers, health practitioners, and patients. As a forum for the entire alternative medicine community, it presents scientific information (pros and cons) on a wide variety of alternative medicine topics.
Website: www.townsendletter.com

Tufts University Health And Nutrition Letter

Tufts Health & Nutrition Letter provides the consumer with honest, reliable, scientifically authoritative health and nutrition advice that not only can be trusted but can have a direct and often immediate effect on their health. The content of this newsletter is based substantially from the research and expertise of the Friedman School of Nutrition Science and Policy.
Website: www.nutritionletter.tufts.edu

University of California, Berkeley Wellness Letter

Berkeley Wellness is an evidence-based wellness information that gives a day-to-day approach to a long and healthful life. It provides positive health and medical tips to help us make decisions that improve our well being, both in mind and in body.
Website: www.berkeleywellness.com

Chapter 69

Directory Of Resources For More CAM Information

Government Agencies That Provide Information About Complementary And Alternative Medicine

Centers for Disease Control and Prevention (CDC)

1600 Clifton Rd.
Atlanta, GA 30333-4027
Toll-Free: 888-232-6348
Website: www.cdc.gov
E-mail: cdcinfo@cdc.gov

Eunice Kennedy Shriver *National Institute of Child Health and Human Development (NICHD)*

NICHD Information Resource Center
P.O. Box 3006
Rockville, MD 20847
Toll-Free: 800-370-2943
Toll-Free TTY: 888-320-6942
Toll-Free Fax: 866-760-5947
Website: www.nichd.nih.gov
E-mail: NICHDInformationResourceCenter@mail.nih.gov

Food and Nutrition Information Center (FNIC)

U.S. National Agricultural Library (NAL)
10301 Baltimore Ave.
Beltsville, MD 20705-2351
Phone: 301-504-5414
Website: www.nal.usda.gov

National Center for Complementary and Integrative Health (NCCIH)

NCCIH Clearinghouse
9000 Rockville Pike
Bethesda, MD 20892
Toll-Free: 888-644-6226
Toll-Free TTY: 866-464-3615
Toll-Free Fax: 866-464-3616
Website: www.nccih.nih.gov
E-mail: info@nccih.nih.gov

About This Chapter: Resources in this chapter were compiled from several sources deemed reliable; all contact information was verified and updated in January 2018.

National Health Information Center (NHIC)

Office of Disease Prevention and Health Promotion (ODPHP), U.S. Department of Health and Human Services (HHS)
1101 Wootton Pkwy
Ste. LL100
Rockville, MD 20852
Fax: 240-453-8281
Website: www.health.gov
E-mail: odphpinfo@hhs.gov

National Institute of Diabetes and Digestive and Kidney Diseases (NIDDK)

National Institutes of Health (NIH)
9000 Rockville Pike
Bethesda, MD 20892
Toll-Free: 800-860-8747
Toll-Free TTY: 866-569-1162
Website: www.niddk.nih.gov
Email: healthinfo@niddk.nih.gov

National Library of Medicine (NLM)

8600 Rockville Pike
Bethesda, MD 20894
Toll-Free: 888-FIND-NLM (888-346-3656)
Phone: 301-594-5983
Website: www.nlm.nih.gov

Office of Cancer Complementary and Alternative Medicine (OCCAM)

National Cancer Institute (NCI)
9609 Medical Center Dr.
Rm. 5-W-136
Rockville, MD 20850
Toll-Free: 800-4-CANCER (800-422-6237)
Phone: 240-276-6595
Toll-Free TTY: 800-332-8615
Fax: 240-276-7888
Website: www.cam.cancer.gov
E-mail: ncioccam1-r@mail.nih.gov

Office of Dietary Supplements (ODS)

National Institutes of Health (NIH)
6100 Executive Blvd.
Rm. 3B01, MSC 7517
Bethesda, MD 20892-7517
Phone: 301-435-2920
Fax: 301-480-1845
Website: www.ods.od.nih.gov
E-mail: ods@nih.gov

U.S. Food and Drug Administration (FDA)

10903 New Hampshire Ave.
Silver Spring, MD 20993
Toll-Free: 888-INFO-FDA (888-463-6332)
Website: www.fda.gov

Private Agencies That Provide Information About Complementary And Alternative Medicine

Academy of Nutrition and Dietetics
120 S. Riverside Plaza
Ste. 2190
Chicago, IL 60606-6995
Toll-Free: 800-877-1600
Phone: 312-899-0040
Fax: 312-899-4873
Website: www.eatright.org
E-mail: acend@eatright.org

Alexander Technique International (ATI)
1692 Massachusetts Ave.
Cambridge, MA 02138
Toll-Free: 888-668-8996
Phone: 617-497-5151
Fax: 617-497-2615
Website: www.alexandertechniqueinternational.com

The American Academy of Allergy, Asthma & Immunology (AAAAI)
555 East Wells St.
Ste. 1100
Milwaukee, WI 53202-3823
Phone: 414-272-6071
Website: www.aaaai.org
E-mail: info@aaaai.org

American Academy of Medical Acupuncture (AAMA)
2512 Artesia Blvd., Ste. 200
Redondo Beach, CA 90278
Phone: 310-379-8261
Website: www.medicalacupuncture.org
E-mail: info@medicalacupuncture.org

American Art Therapy Association (AATA)
4875 Eisenhower Ave., Ste. 240
Alexandria, VA 22304
Toll-Free: 888-290-0878
Phone: 703-548-5860
Fax: 703-783-8468
Website: www.arttherapy.org

American Association of Acupuncture and Oriental Medicine (AAAOM)
P.O. Box 96503 #44114
Washington, DC 20090-6503
Website: www.aaaomonline.org
E-mail: admin@aaaomonline.org

American Association of Colleges of Osteopathic Medicine (AACOM)
7700 Old Georgetown Rd., Ste. 250
Bethesda, MD 20814
Phone: 301-968-4100
Fax: 301-968-4101
Website: www.aacom.org

American Association of Naturopathic Physicians (AANP)

818 18th St. N.W.
Ste. 250
Washington, DC 20006
Toll Free: 866-538-2267
Phone: 202-237-8150
Fax: 202-237-8152
Website: www.naturopathic.org

American Association of Professional Hypnotherapists (AAPH)

1430 Willamette St.
Ste. 47
Eugene, OR 97401-4049
Phone: 458-215-2424
Website: www.aaph.org

American Botanical Council (ABC)

6200 Manor Rd.
Austin, TX 78723
Toll-Free: 800-373-7105
Phone: 512-926-4900
Fax: 512-926-2345
Website: abc.herbalgram.org
E-mail: abc@herbalgram.org

American Cancer Society (ACS)

250 Williams St. N.W.
Atlanta, GA 30303
Toll-Free: 800-227-2345
Website: www.cancer.org

American Chiropractic Association (ACA)

1701 Clarendon Blvd.
Ste. 200
Arlington, VA 22209
Phone: 703-276-8800
Fax: 703-243-2593
Website: www.acatoday.org
E-mail: memberinfo@acatoday.org

American College of Asthma, Allergy, and Immunology (AAAI)

85 W. Algonquin Rd.
Ste. 550
Arlington Heights, IL 60005
Phone: 847-427-1200
Fax: 847-427-9656
Website: www.acaai.org

American Dance Therapy Association (ADTA)

10632 Little Patuxent Pkwy
Ste. 108
Columbia, MD 21044
Phone: 410-997-4040
Fax: 410-997-4048
Website: www.adta.org

American Diabetes Association (ADA)

2451 Crystal Dr.
Ste. 900
Arlington, VA 22202
Toll-Free: 800-DIABETES (800-342-2383)
Website: www.diabetes.org
E-mail: AskADA@diabetes.org

American Herbal Pharmacopoeia (AHP)
P.O. Box 66809
Scotts Valley, CA 95067
Phone: 831-461-6318
Fax: 831-438-2196
Website: www.herbal-ahp.org/index.html
Email: ahp@herbal-ahp.org

American Herbal Products Association (AHPA)
8630 Fenton St.
Ste. 918
Silver Spring, MD 20910
Phone: 301-588-1171
Fax: 301-588-1174
Website: www.ahpa.org
E-mail: ahpa@ahpa.org

American Herbalists Guild (AHG)
P.O. Box 3076
Asheville, NC 28802-3076
Phone: 617-520-4372
Website: www.americanherbalistsguild.com
E-mail: office@americanherbalistsguild.com

American Holistic Health Association (AHHA)
P.O. Box 17400
Anaheim, CA 92817-7400
Phone: 714-779-6152
Website: www.ahha.org
E-mail: mail@ahha.org

American Holistic Medical Association (AHMA)
6919 La Jolla Blvd.
San Diego, CA 92037
Phone: 858-240-9033
Website: www.holisticmedicine.org

American Holistic Nurses Association (AHNA)
2900 S.W. Plass Ct.
Topeka, KS 66611-1980
Toll Free: 800-278-2462
Phone: 785-234-1712
Fax: 785-234-1713
Website: www.ahna.org

American Institute for Preventive Medicine
30445 Northwestern Hwy., Ste. 350
Farmington Hills, MI 48334
Toll-Free: 800-345-2476
Phone: 248-539-1800
Fax: 248-539-1808
Website: healthylife.com
E-mail: aipm@healthylife.com

American Institute of Homeopathy (AIH)
c/o Sandra M. Chase, MD, DHt, Trustee
10418 Whitehead St.
Fairfax, VA 22030
Toll-Free: 888-445-9988
Website: www.homeopathyusa.org
E-mail: admin@homeopathyusa.org

American Massage Therapy Association (AMTA)
500 Davis St.
Ste. 900
Evanston, IL 60201-4695
Toll Free: 877-905-0577
Phone: 847-864-0123
Fax: 847-864-5196
Website: www.amtamassage.org
E-mail: info@amtamassage.org

American Meditation Institute (AMI)
60 Garner Rd.
Averill Park, NY 12018
Phone: 518-674-8714
Website: www.americanmeditation.org
E-mail: info@americanmeditation.org

American Music Therapy Association (AMTA)
8455 Colesville Rd.
Ste. 1000
Silver Spring, MD 20910
Phone: 301-589-3300
Fax: 301-589-5175
Website: www.musictherapy.org
E-mail: info@musictherapy.org

American Osteopathic Association (AOA)
142 East Ontario St.
Chicago, IL 60611
Toll Free: 888-626-9262
Fax: 312-202-8202
Website: www.osteopathic.org
E-mail: crc@osteopathic.org

American Psychiatric Association (APA)
800 Maine Ave. S.W.
Ste. 900
Washington, DC 20024
Phone: 202-559-3900
Website: www.psych.org
E-mail: apa@psych.org

American Psychological Association (APA)
750 First St. N.E.
Washington, DC 20002-4242
Toll-Free: 800-374-2721
Phone: 202-336-5500
TDD/TTY: 202-336-6123
Website: www.apa.org

The American Reflexology Certification Board
2586 Knightsbridge Rd. S.E.
Grand Rapids, MI 49546
Phone: 303-933-6921
Fax: 303-904-0460
Website: www.arcb.net
E-mail: info@arcb.net

American Society for the Alexander Technique (AmSAT)
11 W. Monument Ave.
Ste. 510
Dayton, OH 45402-1233
Toll-Free: 800-473-0620
Phone: 937-586-3732
Website: www.amsatonline.org

American Society of Clinical Hypnosis (ASCH)
140 N. Bloomingdale Rd.
Bloomingdale, IL 60108
Phone: 630-980-4740
Fax: 630-351-8490
Website: www.asch.net
E-mail: info@asch.net

Anxiety Disorders Association of America (ADAA)

8701 Georgia Ave.
Ste. 412
Silver Spring, MD 20910
Phone: 240-485-1001
Fax: 240-485-1035
Website: www.adaa.org

Associated Bodywork and Massage Professionals (ABMP)

25188 Genesee Trail Rd.
Ste. 200
Golden, CO 80401
Toll-Free: 800-458-2267
Toll-Free Fax: 800-667-8260
Website: www.abmp.com
E-mail: expectmore@abmp.com

Association for Applied Psychophysiology and Biofeedback (AAPB)

10200 W. 44th Ave.
Ste. 304
Wheat Ridge, CO 80033
Toll Free: 800-477-8892
Phone: 303-422-8436
Website: www.aapb.org
E-mail: info@aapb.org

Asthma and Allergy Foundation of America (AAFA)

8201 Corporate Dr.
Ste. 1000
Landover, MD 20785
Toll-Free: 800-7-ASTHMA (800-727-8462)
Website: www.aafa.org
E-mail: info@aafa.org

Ayurvedic Institute

11311 Menaul Blvd. N.E.
Albuquerque, NM 87112
Phone: 505-291-9698
Fax: 505-294-7572
Website: www.ayurveda.com

Benson-Henry Institute for Mind Body Medicine (BHI)

Massachusetts General Hospital
55 Fruit St.
Boston, MA 02114
Phone: 617-726-2000
Website: www.massgeneral.org/bhi

The Center for Mind-Body Medicine

5225 Connecticut Ave. N.W.
Ste. 414
Washington, DC 20015
Phone: 202-966-7338
Fax: 202-966-2589
Website: cmbm.org

Center for Spirituality, Theology, and Health

Duke University Medical Center
P.O. Box 3400
Busse Bldg. Ste. 0505
Durham, NC 27710
Phone: 919-681-6633
Fax: 919-684-8569
Website: www.spiritualityandhealth.duke.edu

Center for the Study of Complementary and Alternative Therapies (CSCAT)
University of Virginia School of Medicine
1224 West Main St.
Ste. G113
Charlottesville, VA 22903
Phone: 434-297-4209
Fax: 434-243-9938
Website: www.medicine.virginia.edu

Charlotte Maxwell Complementary Clinic
610 16th St.
Ste. 426
Oakland, CA 94612
Phone: 510-601-7660
Fax: 510-601-7669
Website: www.charlottemaxwell.org

Cleveland Clinic
9500 Euclid Ave.
Cleveland, OH 44195
Toll-Free: 800-223-2273
Website: www.clevelandclinic.org

Duke Integrative Medicine
DUMC P.O. Box 102904
Durham, NC 27710
Toll-Free: 866-313-0959
Phone: 919-660-6826
Website: www.dukeintegrativemedicine.org

Feldenkrais Method of Somatic Education
401 Edgewater Pl., Ste. 600
Wakefield, MA 01880
Phone: 781-876-8935
Fax: 781-645-1322
Website: www.feldenkrais.com

The Food Allergy and Anaphylaxis Network (FAAN)
7925 Jones Branch Dr.
Ste. 1100
McLean, VA 22102
Toll-Free: 800-929-4040
Phone: 703-691-3179
Fax: 703-691-2713
Website: www.foodallergy.org

Guild for Structural Integration (GSI)
65 Enterprise
Aliso Viejo, CA 92656
Toll-Free: 800-447-0150
Phone: 949-715-7449
Fax: 949-715-6931
Website: www.rolfguild.org
E-mail: info@rolfguild.org

Herb Research Foundation
5589 Arapahoe Ave.
Ste. 205
Boulder, CO 80303
Phone: 303-449-2265
Fax: 303-449-7849
Website: www.herbs.org

Institute for Traditional Medicine (ITM)
2017 S.E. Hawthorne Blvd.
Portland, OR 97214
Phone: 503-233-4907
Fax: 503-233-1017
Website: www.itmonline.org

International Center for Reiki Training (ICRT)
21421 Hilltop St.
Unit #28
Southfield, MI 48033
Toll Free: 800-332-8112
Phone: 248-948-8112
Fax: 248-948-9534
Website: www.reiki.org
E-mail: center@reiki.org

International Chiropractic Association (ICA)
6400 Arlington Blvd.
Ste. 800
Falls Church, VA 22042
Toll-Free: 800-423-4690
Phone: 703-528-5000
Fax: 703-528-5023
Website: www.chiropractic.org

International Food Information Council Foundation (IFIC)
1100 Connecticut Ave. N.W., Ste. 430
Washington, DC 20036
Phone: 202-296-6540
Website: www.foodinsight.org
E-mail: info@foodinsight.org

Joslin Diabetes Center
One Joslin Pl.
Boston, MA 02215
Phone: 617-309-2400
Website: www.joslin.org

Micronutrient Information Center (MIC)
Linus Pauling Institute, Oregon State University
307 Linus Pauling Science Center
Corvallis, OR 97331
Phone: 541-737-5075
Fax: 541-737-5077
Website: lpi.orst.edu/infocenter
E-mail: lpi@oregonstate.edu

National Association for Holistic Aromatherapy (NAHA)
P.O. Box 27871
Raleigh, NC 27611-7871
Phone: 919-894-0298
Fax: 919-894-0271
Website: www.naha.org
E-mail: info@naha.org

National Ayurvedic Medical Association (NAMA)
620 Cabrillo Ave.
8605 Santa Monica Blvd., #46789
Los Angeles, CA 90069-4109
Toll-Free: 800-669-8914
Website: www.ayurveda-nama.org
E-mail: nama@ayurvedaNAMA.org

National Center for Homeopathy (NCH)
1120 Rt. 73
Ste. 200
Mount Laurel, NJ 08054
Phone: 856-437-4752
Fax: 856-439-0525
Website: nationalcenterforhomeopathy.org

National Certification Commission for Acupuncture and Oriental Medicine (NCCAOM)

2025 M St. N.W., Ste. 800
Washington, DC 20036
Toll Free: 888-381-1140
Phone: 202-381-1140
Fax: 202-381-1141
Website: www.nccaom.org
E-mail: info@nccaom.org

National Qigong Association (NQA)

P.O. Box 270065
St. Paul, MN 55127
Toll-Free: 888-815-1893
Website: www.nqa.org
E-mail: info@nqa.org

Price-Pottenger Nutrition Foundation (PPNF)

7890 Bdwy.
Lemon Grove, CA 91945
Toll-Free: 800-366-3748
Phone: 619-462-7600
Fax: 619-433-3136
Website: price-pottenger.org
E-mail: info@price-pottenger.org

Qigong Association of America (AQA)

27133 Forest Springs Ln.
Corvallis, OR 97330
Toll-Free: 888-9-QIGONG (888-974-4664)
Website: www.qi.org

Qigong Institute (QI)

617 Hawthorne Ave.
Los Altos, CA 94024
Website: www.qigonginstitute.org
E-mail: qi@qigonginstitute.org

Reflexology Association of America (RAA)

14471 81st Ave.
Dyer, IN 46311
Phone: 980-234-0159
Website: www.reflexology-usa.org
E-mail: infoRAA@reflexology-usa.org

Rolf Institute of Structural Integration

5055 Chaparral Ct.
Ste. 103
Boulder, CO 80301
Phone: 303-449-5903
Fax: 303-449-5978
Website: www.rolf.org

Stanford Center for Integrative Medicine

211 Quarry Rd.
Second Fl.
Palo Alto, CA 94304
Phone: 650-498-5566
Fax: 650-498-5640
Website: stanfordhealthcare.org

Sutter Pacific Medical Foundation

Institute for Health and Healing (IHH)
2300 California St.
Ste. 202
San Francisco, CA 94115
Phone: 415-600-3503
Website: www.sutterpacific.org

University of Arizona Center for Integrative Medicine (AzCIM)

Arizona Center for Integrative Medicine
P.O. Box 245153
Tucson, AZ 85724-5153
Website: integrativemedicine.arizona.edu

University of California, San Francisco (UCSF) Osher Center for Integrative Medicine

1545 Divisadero St.
Fourth Fl.
San Francisco, CA 94115-3010
Phone: 415-353-7700
Fax: 415-353-7358
Website: www.osher.ucsf.edu
E-mail: ocim@ocim.ucsf.edu

Index

Index

Page numbers that appear in *Italics* refer to tables or illustrations. Page numbers that have a small 'n' after the page number refer to citation information shown as Notes. Page numbers that appear in **Bold** refer to information contained in boxes within the chapters.

A

B

C

D

E

F

G

H

I

J

N

O

P

Q

R

S

T

U

V

W

X

Y

Z